Girlfriends on the Go

Suzie Roberts

CFI
Springville, Utah

No part of this book may be reproduced in any form whatsoever, whether by graphic, visual, electronic, film, microfilm, tape recording, or any other means, without prior written permission of the publisher, except in the case of brief passages embodied in critical reviews and articles.

ISBN 13: 978-1-59955-015-2

Published by CFI, an imprint of Cedar Fort, Inc., 2373 W. 700 S., Springville, UT, 84663
Distributed by Cedar Fort, Inc. www.cedarfort.com

LIBRARY OF CONGRESS CATALOGING-IN-PUBLICATION DATA

Roberts, Suzie.
  Girlfriends on the go : a busy mom's guide to make-ahead meals / Suzie Roberts.
    p. cm.
  ISBN 978-1-59955-015-2
  1. Make-ahead cookery. 2. Cookery (Frozen foods) I. Title.

  TX652.R6357 2007
  641.5'55--dc22

                          2007000589

Cover and page design by Nicole Williams
Edited by Annaliese B. Cox
Cover design © 2007 by Lyle Mortimer

Printed in China

10 9 8 7 6 5 4 3 2 1

Printed on acid-free paper

"What's for dinner?" So you say

It's been another crazy day.

Soccer, piano, homework, and more,

I didn't have time to go to the store.

"Let's order out!" The kids say with a grin.

"Pizza again?" says Dad with a cringe.

Then what should we have? Something homemade for sure.

None of this stuff in a box from the store!

"Never you fear," I say with a sigh,

The freezer is full of meals to the sky.

How 'bout lasagna or chicken sweet n' sour?

"Hurry quick, put it in, I have book club in an hour!"

Now there's one more problem left to be solved,

Whose turn to clean up after everyone involved?

"We'll clear our dishes," the kids say and dash.

Mom grabs her book and is out with a flash.

Dad looks around—all these empty seats,

A familiar sight after everyone eats.

It's time for the game; Dad's a huge football fan

But not 'till he throws out the disposable pan.

Table of Contents

"The Make-Ahead Meal Group has been such a great thing for my family. I own a childcare center with over 200 children and I am currently PTA president for an elementary school. With my life being so full, I want to spend every minute with my children as possible. Being part of a casserole club has helped me with that. Dinner isn't stressful, and we can enjoy a home-cooked meal. I think that without the Make-Ahead Meal Group, many of our meals would be fast food, which isn't healthy or cheap."

Ty Singleton, PTA President, Business owner

"The Make-Ahead Meal Group has simplified my life and has also saved it at times! I always know that there will be hot meal on the table for my family. I struggle with being creative and trying new things for dinner, but this group has solved both of these problems. We love it and can't imagine life without the group!"

Marci Satterthwaite, PTA President, City Council Person

Acknowledgments

I express my gratitude to an awesome friend, Kristen Taylor, for her advice and for letting me "pick her brain" where mine left off. I appreciate her time and talent in editing this book.

This cookbook would also not have happened without the help of a great author and friend, Josi Kilpack. Thank you, Josi, for your suggestions and editing.

I extend a sincere thanks to another fabulous friend, Nancy Moyle, for her editing expertise and encouragement.

Thank you, Dave, for being my food critic, for believing in me and encouraging me, and for being the wonderful husband and father that you are. I love you!

To my children, Kyra, Kuen, Tatem, and Bryson: If it weren't for you, there would be no need for me to use my talents and ideas in trying to make our crazy life run smoothly. Thanks for your fun personalities! I love you!

Thanks to all my "Casserole Club" members, past and present, who have been willing to share their talents with other families. Thanks for going through all the experimental stages of the Make-Ahead Meal Group in order to make this book possible.

All About Make-Ahead Meals

Introduction

It's one of those days. You know—*those* days. The phone is ringing off the hook, the kids need help with their homework, your husband is working late, you have a PTA meeting in an hour and still have to pick kids up from soccer practice. Then you think about dinner. Dinner? Okay, here are the quick and easy choices: pizza, pizza, or pizza. Okay, kids . . . how about pizza?

As you fall into bed later that night and analyze your day, you realize that all was running smoothly, one challenge at a time, until 5 p.m. Dinnertime came and you weren't prepared, so everything else seemed to fall apart. Does it seem to be this way more often than not? Do you want it to be different?

This book is tailored to the mom who does it all—the mom with a busy life and busy children but who wants to have peaceful, fulfilling family time every night at the dinner table; the mom who wants to feed her family home-cooked meals but wants less time planning and preparing those meals.

Whether you want to start a Make-Ahead Meal Group or participate in one or just prepare Make-Ahead Meals for your own family, this book is the tool to help you achieve that goal. It will assist you in planning and preparing Make-Ahead Meals that have been tried and tested by actual Make-Ahead Meal Groups. We've picked only the best meals for you and your family.

Good luck in your endeavors to simplify life, save time and money, enjoy more family time, make some great friends, and be treated to a variety of delicious home-cooked meals.

What Is a Make-Ahead Meal Group?

A Make-Ahead Meal Group is a group of people who prepare and freeze a designated number of the same meal of their choice in the convenience of their own home. Then they get together to exchange dishes so that each member of the group takes home that same number of various meals. It is designed to save time, money, and stress by spending one afternoon making one meal in bulk rather than spending the time every night to prepare a home-cooked meal for your family. This book will give you the tricks of the trade along with many tried and true recipes to help you simplify dinnertime in your own home.

How to Start Your Own Make-Ahead Meal Group

Invite people to join your group:

Think of all the moms you know who could use a little simplifying in their lives—maybe your neighbor, friend, sister-in-law, or fellow soccer moms. Think of those moms who are dependable, good cooks, and have healthy homes (clean kitchen habits). These are the type of people you should look for so that you feel good about where your meals are coming from. You may also suggest that your members get a food handler's permit. It isn't necessary, but it's a good idea for food safety. (Call your local health department for information.)

Make some rules and guidelines:

It is very important that everyone in your group knows exactly what is expected of them so that everyone can do their part. (See page 9 for sample guidelines.) You'll want to have a meeting before your group starts so that everyone can discuss and decide what works best for your specific group. The issues to address are:

- **How many** people each meal must feed. For example, many groups set the amount at 6 adult servings, and if the meal is in a casserole dish, require that the dish be 9×13 inches in size. For those families that don't eat quite that much, it is perfect for leftovers and to send with your husband to work the next day.

- **Decide what** preferences you will cater to. For instance, some groups prefer boneless, skinless chicken breasts. Also, you will need to address food allergies. Many groups find it is easier to not have any food allergy guidelines. However, if the majority of group members prefer low-fat or all-chicken meals, then make it a group requirement.

- **Decide a** time and place to exchange. In case someone can't make it to the exchange on the specified day, it is helpful to make the exchange at a member's house that has extra freezer space. Then those who can't make it to the exchange can deliver their meals the day before and have somewhere to keep it frozen until the other members pick up the meals. Coolers with ice also work well if any group members will be picking up the meals shortly after the exchange.

- **Decide when,** where, and how often to exchange meals. Choosing a specific day of each month will help your members always know when it is coming and can plan around it. Exchanges can be bi-monthly or however often your group wants it to be. Choosing a date such as the second Friday of every month is often easier than, for example, the 10th of each month, so that you avoid hitting the weekends.

- **Set an** approximate price range. Otherwise, someone may spend $30 on their meals and someone else may spend $150. A good average is $75. It is feasible to spend less, especially if you watch the sales, but encourage your members not to go over the budget and to choose meals within the budget.

- **Have group** members bring copies of their recipes to each exchange. A full sheet of paper can be kept in a binder specifically for Make-Ahead Meal recipes. Or exchange 3×5 recipe cards to fit in your recipe file. Do whatever works best for group members. Each member should put her name and phone number on her recipe in case other members have questions about it. Side dish suggestions are a helpful addition to each recipe.

- **Decide who** is in charge. Your group may want to take turns making reminder calls. Some groups may not even need reminder calls, but it is often appreciated. Most groups choose one person as the president, so to say, and she does all the reminding and finds people to fill vacant spots. This could change every year if desired.

After the meeting, send group members a welcome letter or email that includes all the guidelines decided by the group. Make sure each member receives one. This is especially nice for new members who join later. See a sample guideline letter on page 9.

Welcome to the Make-Ahead Meal Group!

Here are the guidelines:

• **You will** be required to make and freeze 10 meals to exchange with our group.

• **Try to** spend around or below $75 for all costs.

• **Your meal** should feed 6 adults. (If item is in a pan, please use a 9×13.)

• **You will** need to package your meal either in freezer bags or disposable aluminum pans.

• **Write on** your packaging with permanent marker what the meal is, the basic instructions, and the date (example: Chicken Casserole, 350° for 30 min, 02/02/07). You will probably have to pull the meal out of the freezer ahead of time so that it can thaw. Write the cook time that should be used once the meal is thawed.

• **Please only** make meals that you and your family have tried and enjoy. Don't experiment on the group!

• **If you** are stumped about what to cook and what freezes well, there is a great book that has all the tips and recipes that you'll need. It is called *Girlfriends on the Go: A Busy Mom's Guide to Make-Ahead Meals* by Suzie Roberts.

• **Type up** each of your recipes on a full sheet of paper as well as suggestions for what vegetables or side dishes to serve with the meal. We want to be able to put each recipe in its own sheet protector so that we can put together a binder specifically for Make-Ahead Meal recipes. Also, write your name on the recipe page so that we remember who made the meal.

• **We want** everyone to have fun. Obviously your family is not going to love every meal, but hopefully they will enjoy the majority and that will make it all worthwhile. The most important thing is to take some stress out of your day so that you can spend more time with your family doing fun things, not cooking and cleaning!

• **Also, pay** attention to your grocery and dining-out budget so that you can see the money you've saved.

Our next meal exchange will be on _____ at _____'s house at _____.

Her address is _____.

Please bring your meals already frozen. Plan ahead! If you cannot make it to the exchange, please drop off the meals in a cooler (with ice) prior to the exchange. If you are not prepared, each person will keep their meal until you deliver your meal and pick up theirs from each group member. We will meet every second Friday to exchange and tell about our dish. It shouldn't take more than 45 minutes.

Please call if you have any questions!

Frequently Asked Questions about Make-Ahead Meal Groups

How long does it take to prepare 10 meals?

It depends on the meal. It usually takes 2–4 hours. We have found that it works best in shifts. For instance, one day you can cook all the meat and the next day assemble the rest. It may sound like a long time, but those ten days that you don't have to take the time and have the mess of preparing meals makes it worth it. With good planning you can save time and frustration by preparing your meals when your kids are asleep or at school.

How does a Make-Ahead Meal Group save you money?

Let me count the ways . . .

- **First, you** go to the grocery store less often. Do you ever go to the store for milk and bread and end up coming out with 10 other items you didn't need? The less often you visit the store, the less money you will spend.

- **Your shopping** list for Make-Ahead Meals is simple. You don't need a list of items for 10 different meals. Instead, you buy 10 of the same thing. Simple is good.

- **You can** plan your meals around what's on sale. If ground beef is on sale, choose a recipe for that month that calls for ground beef.

- **You'll eat** out less. Fridays and Saturdays are great times for Make-Ahead Meals because those are usually the days that you don't feel like cooking. Know your family and pull a meal out of the freezer on days you know you won't have time to cook.

- **You have** less waste. Since you don't purchase ingredients for several different meals, perishable ingredients don't go bad before you have a chance to use them.

- **You can** purchase items in bulk. Watch those sales or shop at a warehouse store (like Costco). It's cheaper and leaves less packaging to throw away.

What if someone quits?

If someone quits, try to fill the spot at as soon as possible. If you are not able to fill that spot in time for the next exchange, you have several options:

1. On the exchange day, tell everyone in your group to take their extra meal home with them.

2. Have everyone exchange their extra meal among themselves so that they take two of another meal home instead of two of their own.

3. Give the extra meals to someone who needs it that month, such as someone who just had surgery or a baby or someone whose spouse is on military duty.

4. Another option is to have a substitute that is willing to participate when someone is unable to do it.

How does a Make-Ahead Meal Group save you time?

If you spend 4 hours making 10 meals, including prep and cleanup, you will save yourself as much as 16 hours a month. How? If you were to make a meal every night for 10 nights, you would take approximately 15 minutes to decide what you'll have, 30 minutes to run to the store to get the ingredients you're missing, and 45 minutes to chop, boil, brown, marinate, simmer, and assemble. Then there are all the dishes, pots, bowls, cutting boards, utensils, and appliances that you used in the preparation process that you need to wash, dry, and put away. That takes you at least another 20 minutes. As you are doing all of this, of course there are at least 15 minutes of interruptions. You don't always realize that it takes so much time to prepare a meal every night, but you will realize the extra time on those 10 nights that you don't have to.

How many people should be in the group?

Each group can decide for themselves how many meals to make. Most groups find that 10 meals is usually a good amount to exchange each month. That way, you can still fix your family favorites on some days and have left-overs other days. I personally have found that the best use of the meals is to eat them on your busiest days. Maybe Tuesdays are T-ball games and piano lessons. Use a Make-Ahead Meal on those days. I almost always use Make-Ahead Meals on Fridays since that is the day I have found that I don't feel like cooking and would usually order pizza. For many people, Sundays are good for Make-Ahead Meals because it takes less effort to put a nice Sunday dinner on the table—and much less cleanup.

What if we have picky eaters?

Obviously there are going to be some meals that members of your family just don't like. Before I started the Make-Ahead Meal Group, I could count on one hand the things my 6-year-old son would eat. However, I felt it was important for him to learn to try new things and believed that if he would try new things, he would like them. Since we always had a variety of food and didn't always have the same old meals that I knew all my kids would eat, he had to learn to try many new things. A year later, he would eat any kind of chicken and some casseroles. For me, that has been the biggest reward from the Make-Ahead Meal Group. Since then, I have had a 1-year-old who loves any food I put in front of him. I believe that this acceptance of foods is from having a variety of meals from a young age.

What are other benefits of a Make-Ahead Meal Group?

- **Someone else's** cooking: Sometimes food just tastes better when someone else prepares it—not because you're not a good cook, but because you don't have to cook it.

- **Variety:** You don't always have the same old meals. Of course, your family has their favorites, and the days you don't use a Make-Ahead Meal are perfect for those family favorites. People often find meals they'd never considered making have become a new favorite.

- **Sick Days:** Mom doesn't get a day off when she's sick—it's nice to have one less thing to do on those days.

- **Dad's turn** to cook: Dad will love the Make-Ahead Meals on those nights he's in charge. With the instructions written right on the package, he can just put a meal in the oven when it's his turn to cook.

- **Serving others:** When a friend or a loved one is having a hard time, it's nice to have a meal that you can easily share. Some people in our Make-Ahead Meal Group choose to make an extra meal each month, and we get together and take the extra meals to someone in need that month, such as a family whose mom or dad is on military duty, a mom who just had a baby, someone having financial troubles, someone who has had a death in the family or a serious illness, and so forth. It's funny how a few meals can take a large burden off someone in need.

What is the best way to thaw our Make-Ahead Meals?

For best results, let frozen meals thaw in the refrigerator for 24 hours. For those of us who don't think that far in advance, here are some other tips:

- **If cooking** directly from frozen, as a rule of thumb, bump up the temperature 50° higher than the recipe states, and double the time. Generally, this is ample time to cook your frozen meal. You will need to check it periodically to make sure you are on target.

What if someone quits? (cont.)

5. Have someone in the group make an extra set of meals and receive double meals that month.

6. If it is early enough, you could call your group and tell them to make one less meal that month. But keep in mind that some members may have already prepared their meals.

Flash Freezing

Sometimes you will need to flash freeze items such as meatballs or chicken pockets —anything you will put in a freezer bag in which you don't want individual items to stick together.

To flash freeze, place the items on a cookie sheet and put it in the freezer. As soon as they are no longer soft to the touch they are ready to be placed in a bag and returned to the freezer.

• **If you** will be out of the house all day, a slow cooker meal is perfect. You can put it in your slow cooker in the morning and it will be ready at dinnertime. If there are no slow cooker meals in your freezer, your time-delay cook on your oven is also a wonderful tool. Place your meal in the oven at your convenience. Set your bake time about 1½ times the amount called for in the recipe, and set your temperature 25°–50° higher. Your meal will have time to partially thaw in the oven until it starts to cook at the designated time. What a good feeling to walk in to the scent of a nice home-cooked meal after a hard day's work.

Make-Ahead Meal Tips

As you are trying to make your life simpler, read all the tips I've learned through years of experience with Make-Ahead Meals. This will save you from having to experiment yourself. I have made it as simple as possible to make it less time consuming and more productive for you. Remember, the people who need Make-Ahead Meals are the ones who don't have time for the small details, just the cold, hard . . . meal!

What to freeze your meals in:

Freezer Bags:

• **If at** all possible, freeze your meals in freezer bags. They are the cheapest way to go. Many soups, sauces, and non-layered type casseroles can be frozen in a gallon-size freezer bag.

• **Squeeze as** much air out of the bag as you can. The less air, the less freezer taste and freezer burn your meal will have.

• **Label the** freezer bag *before* you freeze it.

• **Once filled,** lay your bag flat in the freezer. It will freeze quicker that way and take up less room in the freezer. Don't stack meals on top of each other until after they are frozen so that they can freeze properly in the middle.

Disposable Pans:

• **Disposable aluminum** pans work great for anything that can't be put in a freezer bag.

• **Make sure** you cover the dish tightly with foil. You may also wish to use a double layer of foil or freezer foil to protect your meals even more. If the meal is tomato based, cover with plastic wrap and then foil. The acid from the tomatoes can eat away the foil.

Foods that may not freeze well:

• **If you** are making a meal that uses flour tortillas, such as enchiladas, freeze the enchiladas separate from the sauce. Put the sauce in a quart-size freezer bag and freeze along with the meal. Otherwise, your tortillas may get very mushy.

• **If your** meal calls for cooked rice or pasta, undercook it, or it will get mushy from freezing and thawing.

• **Raw potatoes** or squashes do not freeze well. If you are using potatoes or vegetables that need to be cooked before freezing, undercook them so they don't get mushy. Potatoes tend to get mushy anyway. If possible, replace potatoes with frozen hash browns, which have been commercially prepared for freezing.

• **You can** purchase disposable aluminum pans in bulk at wholesale stores. They end up being about 25 cents apiece. It is so nice to just throw away the mess, instead of soaking and scrubbing a pan.

Cooking Meat in Bulk

When you are preparing meals for a group, it is easier to cook your meat in bulk. Here are some ways to simplify this process.

• **Ground Beef:** Crumble 3 to 4 lbs. on a large cookie sheet with sides. Place in a preheated oven at 425° and bake for 20 minutes or until meat is no longer pink. Make sure you use extra-lean or extra-extra lean for this process unless you use a casserole dish with taller sides. Otherwise the grease may drip over the edge. Pull out of the oven when done. Place meat in a colander under hot water. Rinse off extra grease as you use a spatula to crumble the meat.

• **Another way** to cook ground beef in bulk is to place in boiling water in a stockpot and boil until no longer pink. Then, rinse in a colander as well.

• **Chicken:** A large slow cooker will do 10–12 chicken breasts at a time. Place them in the slow cooker with 1 cup of water and cook on medium or high for 2–3 hours (longer if you want to shred it–shorter if you want it whole or to cube it). You can also cook it on low overnight in a slow cooker. Anything you can do while you sleep is a great way to multi-task! Such a motherly thing to do!

• **Roasts:** Use a large slow cooker for 1–2 roasts, or even better, use a roaster oven to do 5–6 at a time. Cook on medium overnight. When you wake up, they are ready to shred.

Make-Ahead Meal Icons

The exclamation mark icon will alert you to tips and tricks that make freezing meals easier.

The shopping cart icon will show you a list of ingredients you will need in order to make a Make-Ahead Meal for 10 families.

The snowflake icon appears with each recipe to give you directions for freezing the meal.

Foods that may not freeze well (cont.):

• **Sauces with** sour cream, cream cheese, and cream freeze fine. Depending on the ratio of cream in the sauce, you may need to whisk sauce after re-heating since it may separate slightly after freezing.

The Process

Yes, there can be some method to the madness.

1. After you decide on the meal you want to prepare, check your pantry. Most of the main ingredients called for will probably need to be purchased, but you may already have the spices or other small ingredients. However, don't assume you have enough. You may think you definitely have garlic powder, but if your recipe calls for 1 teaspoon, you will need 10 teaspoons. Nothing is worse than being up to your elbows assembling 10 meals and realizing that you're short one ingredient.

2. After shopping and making sure you have all the ingredients, decide on the pre-meal details. Is it a meal in which the meat needs to be browned, cooked, shredded, or cubed? See our section on cooking meat in bulk for tips on streamlining that process.

3. When you're getting ready to prepare the meals, get everything out and set in sections around your kitchen, placing each ingredient in order as it is used in the recipe.

  • **Open all** the items in cans or packages before you start. It saves time and mess. Also, have packaging labeled and ready to fill so that once finished assembling you can place the prepared meal directly into the freezer.

4. You can choose one of two ways to assemble. If the meal has to be mixed in a bowl, it is easier to mix each meal separately, and then place in the appropriate freezing container.

  • **For instance,** if you are making a soup, go down the line and place all the ingredients in the bowl, mix up, and pour into a freezer bag. If it is a soup that has to cooked first, you could possibly double or triple the batch in a stockpot to save time. If your meal is something such as a layered casserole, you may want to do it assembly style.

• **Place all** the pans out on the table. Prepare the first layer for all 10 meals, place in pan, and move on to the second ingredient. This is very quick and easy.

5. Do not stack meals on top of each other in the freezer before they are completely frozen. Stacking makes it hard for the center to freeze in a timely manner.

Soup Recipes

Soups freeze well, and nothing tastes better on a chilly evening.

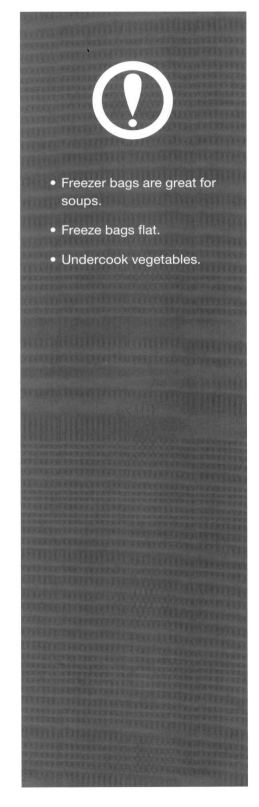

- Freezer bags are great for soups.

- Freeze bags flat.

- Undercook vegetables.

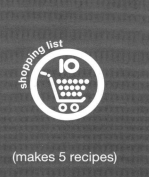

(makes 5 recipes)

- 5 pkgs. frozen broccoli (Abt. 80 oz.)

- 30 carrots

- 20 celery stalks

- 5 medium onions

- 15 cubes butter or margarine

- 7½ cups flour

- 100–120 chicken bouillon cubes

- 5 (16 oz) containers Cheez Whiz or Velveeta cheese

Cheddar Broccoli Soup

(This recipe will make enough for 2 families.)
Breadsticks are always nice to dip in a creamy soup.

1 (16 oz.) pkg. frozen broccoli
6 carrots, sliced
4 stalks of celery, sliced
1 medium onion, chopped
3 cubes butter or margarine
1½ cups flour
10 cups water
10–12 chicken bouillon cubes (to taste)
1 (16 oz.) container Cheez Whiz or Velveeta cheese

Steam vegetables until almost tender. In a separate bowl, microwave butter or margarine until melted. Stir in flour and mix until smooth. In a large saucepan, dissolve bouillon cubes in boiling water. Add a cup of bouillon water to the butter and flour and whisk together. Then add to boiling water and stir. Add drained vegetables to soup. Add Cheez Whiz or Velveeta cheese. Stir until melted. If freezing, see directions below. Otherwise, serve when hot.

Freezing directions: Cool, then put in a freezer bag. Lay flat in freezer.

Chili

(This recipe will make enough for 2 families.)
Easy and satisfying—serve with cornbread and a green salad.

2 lbs. ground beef, browned and drained
2 quarts stewed tomatoes
1 pint salsa
30 oz. chili beans, drained
15 oz. kidney beans, drained
15 oz. pinto beans, drained
1 red bell pepper, chopped
1 green bell pepper, chopped
1 onion, chopped
4 Tbsp. brown sugar
salt to taste
cheddar cheese

Mix all ingredients together. If freezing, see directions below. Otherwise, cook in large slow cooker 3–6 hours. To serve, top with shredded cheese.

 Freezing directions: Divide in half. Pour into gallon-size freezer bags. Include some shredded cheese with this meal.

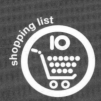

shopping list

(makes 5 recipes)

- 10 lbs. ground beef

- 10 quarts stewed tomatoes

- 5 pints salsa

- 5 large cans chili beans

- 5 (15 oz.) cans kidney beans

- 5 (15 oz.) cans pinto beans

- 5 red bell peppers

- 5 green bell peppers

- 5 onions

- 1¼ cups brown sugar

- 5 lbs. cheddar cheese

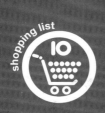

shopping list

- 15 lbs. boneless, skinless chicken breasts
- 5 large onions
- 5 tsp. garlic powder
- Abt. 1 cup butter
- 20 chicken bouillon cubes
- Abt. ¼ cup ground cumin
- 5 quarts half and half
- 5 lbs. shredded Monterey Jack cheese
- 10 (15 oz) cans creamed corn
- 10 (4 oz.) cans chopped green chilies
- 2½ tsp. hot sauce (Tabasco)

10 bags tortilla chips

Mexican Chicken Corn Chowder

This mild, south-of-the-border taste will make your taste buds say "gracias"!

1½ lbs. boneless, skinless chicken breasts
½ cup chopped onion
½ tsp. garlic powder
3 Tbsp. butter
2 chicken bouillon cubes
1 cup hot water
1 tsp. ground cumin
2 cups half and half
2 cups shredded Monterey Jack cheese
1 (15 oz.) can creamed corn
1 (4 oz.) can chopped green chilies
¼ tsp. hot sauce (Tabasco)
1 bag tortilla chips

In large saucepan, brown chicken, onion, garlic, and butter. Dissolve bouillon in hot water and add to chicken. Then add cumin and bring to a boil. Reduce heat, cover, and simmer for 5 minutes. Add remaining ingredients. Cook until cheese melts. If freezing, see directions below. Otherwise, serve topped with crushed tortilla chips.

Freezing directions: Pour into a freezer bag and freeze. Include a bag of tortilla chips with the meal.

Minestrone Soup

Spice up a regular can of minestrone soup and serve with a crusty bread.

1 lb. ground beef
¼ tsp. seasoned salt
¼ tsp. onion salt
1 tsp. dried onions
2 (10 oz.) cans minestrone soup
1 (15 oz.) can pork and beans
1 (15 oz.) can black beans
2 soup cans water

Brown ground beef with salts and dried onions in a large saucepan. Drain. Add the rest of the ingredients. If freezing, see directions below. Otherwise, simmer 20–60 minutes.

- 10 lbs. ground beef
- 2½ tsp. seasoned salt
- 2½ tsp onion salt
- 3 Tbsp. + 1 tsp. dried onions
- 20 cans minestrone soup
- 10 (15 oz.) cans pork and beans
- 10 (15 oz.) cans black beans

Freezing directions: Pour into a gallon-size freezer bag. Seal and freeze.

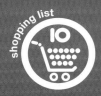

shopping list
10

- 10 lbs. ground beef

- 5 large onions

- 20 large carrots

- 3 bunches celery

- 10 (15 oz.) cans diced tomatoes

- 10 (15 oz.) cans kidney beans

- 20 (15 oz.) cans beef broth

- 10 tsp. oregano

- 5 tsp. pepper

- Abt. ⅓ cup fresh chopped parsley

- 5 tsp. hot sauce (Tabasco)

- 1 jar spaghetti sauce

- 10 small pkgs. shell pasta

Pasta Fagioli Soup

Taste familiar? Popular Italian restaurants serve this same soup.

1 lb. ground beef, browned and drained
1 small onion, chopped
1 cup grated carrots
1 cup diced celery
1 (15 oz.) can diced tomatoes
1 (15 oz.) can kidney beans, drained and rinsed
2 (15 oz.) cans beef broth
1 tsp. oregano
½ tsp. pepper
2 tsp. fresh parsley, chopped
½ tsp. hot sauce (Tabasco)
1 jar spaghetti sauce
1 small bag shell pasta

Place all ingredients in a large saucepan. If freezing, see directions below. Otherwise, simmer until vegetables are tender (30–45 minutes).

Freezing directions: Freeze in gallon-size freezer bags.

Taco Soup

A classic! Kids love eating tacos in a bowl.

1 lb. ground beef, browned and drained
1 (15 oz.) can stewed tomatoes
1 (10 oz.) can tomato soup
1 (10 oz.) can vegetable soup
1 (15 oz.) can corn, drained
1 (15 oz.) can kidney beans, drained and rinsed
¾ cup salsa
1 cup water
2 Tbsp. taco seasoning
2 Tbsp. chili powder

Mix all ingredients together. If freezing, see directions below. Otherwise, place in a large saucepan and cook until hot. Or heat in slow cooker on low for 3 hours. To serve, pour over crushed corn chips and top with sour cream and shredded cheese.

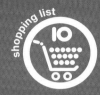

shopping list

- 10 lbs. ground beef
- 10 cans stewed tomatoes
- 10 cans tomato soup
- 10 cans vegetable soup
- 10 cans corn
- 10 cans kidney beans
- Abt. 2 quarts salsa
- Abt. 5 pkgs. taco seasoning
- 1¼ cups chili powder
- 10 small bags corn chips
- 10 small tubs sour cream
- 5 lbs. cheese

Freezing directions: Pour into a gallon-size freezer bag and freeze. Include a bag of corn chips, a carton of sour cream, and some shredded cheese with this meal. (Do not freeze sour cream.)

shopping list

10

- 10 (16 oz.) cans refried beans

- 10 (15 oz.) cans black beans

- 10 (14 oz.) cans chicken broth

- 2 quarts salsa

- 5 (16 oz.) bags frozen corn

- Abt. 10 lbs. boneless, skinless chicken breasts

- Abt. 5 lbs. shredded cheddar cheese

- 5 bags tortilla chips

- 10 small containers sour cream

Tortilla Soup

Adjust the heat in this soup by using mild, medium, or hot salsa.

1 (16 oz.) can refried beans
1 (15 oz.) can black beans, rinsed and drained
1 (14 oz.) can chicken broth
1½ cups frozen corn
¾ cup chunky salsa
1½ cups cooked chicken, cubed
½ cup water
2 cups shredded cheddar cheese
tortilla chips
dollop of sour cream

Combine all ingredients except for the cheese, chips, and sour cream. If freezing, see directions below. Otherwise, simmer for 30 minutes. Crush some tortilla chips in the bottom of the bowls. Add soup and top with sour cream and cheese.

Freezing directions: Place in a gallon-size freezer bag and freeze. Divide a bag of tortilla chips into 2 bags. Put cheese in a freezer bag and include 1 small container of sour cream with each meal. (Do not freeze sour cream.)

Beef Recipes

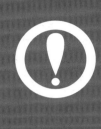

- See page 16 for tips on cooking beef in bulk.

- Ground beef is a great thing to watch the sales for.

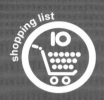

(makes 5 recipes)

- 10 lbs. ground beef

- 5 envelopes chili seasoning mix

- 5 (8 oz.) cans tomato sauce

- 5 cans kidney beans

- 5 cans cream of chicken soup

- 5 lbs. Velveeta cheese

- 3 (16 oz.) pkgs. frozen chopped broccoli

- Abt. 30 lbs. potatoes

- 10 (8 oz.) cartons sour cream

- 10 small pkgs. bacon bits

- 3 bunches green onions

- Abt. 4 lbs. shredded cheddar cheese

Baked Potato Bar

(This recipe will make enough for 2 families.)
Looking for something different? These potatoes are fun and delicious.

Chili:
1 lb. ground beef, browned and drained
1 envelope chili seasoning mix
1 (8 oz.) can tomato sauce
½ cup water
1 can kidney beans, drained

Cheese and broccoli sauce:
1 can cream of chicken soup
1 lb. Velveeta cheese
1–2 cups frozen chopped broccoli

Toppings:
sour cream
bacon bits
green onions
shredded cheese

Chili: Mix all ingredients. Simmer 15 minutes.

Sauce: Heat in a saucepan on medium until melted.

If freezing, see directions below. Otherwise, scrub 8–10 potatoes. Wrap in foil and pierce several times with a fork. Bake at 400° for 1 hour. Top potato with chili or cheese sauce and your choice of toppings.

Freezing directions: The chili and cheese sauce recipes are enough for 2 meals. Divide the chili and cheese sauce in half and place in quart-size freezer bags. Include with this meal 8–10 potatoes, a carton of sour cream, bacon bits, green onions, and 1½ cups shredded cheese. (Do not freeze sour cream.)

Beef and Bean Burritos

The spaghetti sauce adds a surprisingly good flavor to these homemade burritos.

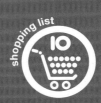

1–1½ lbs. ground beef, browned
¼ cup chopped onion
1 garlic clove, minced
½ Tbsp. chili powder
½ Tbsp. cumin
salt and pepper to taste
1 (8 oz.) can tomato sauce
8 large flour tortillas
1 (16 oz.) can refried beans
1 jar spaghetti sauce
1 cup shredded cheese (cheddar or Monterey Jack)

In a saucepan, mix together browned ground beef, onion, and garlic. Add chili powder, cumin, and other seasonings. Stir in tomato sauce and simmer for 10 minutes. Add refried beans; cook and stir until well blended. Cool completely.

Warm tortillas in microwave for 30 seconds to soften. Place ½–¾ cup of meat mixture on each tortilla. Fold sides of tortilla in and roll up. If freezing, see directions below. Otherwise, place seam-side down in a baking dish and cover with spaghetti sauce and cheese. Bake at 350° for 30 minutes or until hot and bubbly.

Freezing directions: Flash freeze the burritos, and then wrap individually and return to freezer. You can just heat burritos in the microwave and eat separately with salsa and sour cream or bake as directed above with the spaghetti sauce and cheese. Do not freeze with the sauce on them already. The tortillas will get mushy. Include the spaghetti sauce and shredded cheese with this meal.

shopping list

- 10–15 lbs. ground beef
- 5 large onions
- 10 cloves garlic
- 5 Tbsp. chili powder
- 5 Tbsp. cumin
- 10 (8 oz.) cans tomato sauce
- 5 (30 oz.) cans refried beans
- 8 pkgs. large tortillas
- 10 jars spaghetti sauce
- 3 lbs. shredded cheese

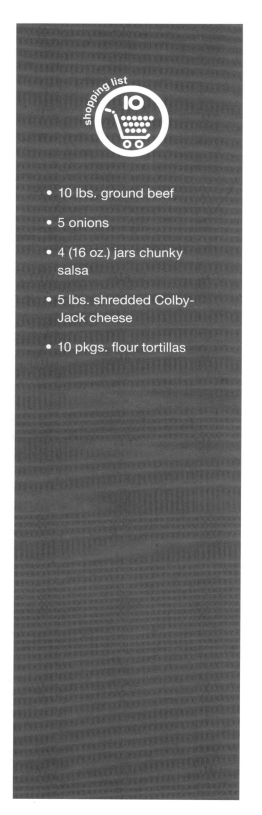

- 10 lbs. ground beef
- 5 onions
- 4 (16 oz.) jars chunky salsa
- 5 lbs. shredded Colby-Jack cheese
- 10 pkgs. flour tortillas

Beef and Cheese Quesadillas

Tortillas freeze well as long as they are kept separate from the liquids in your recipe.

1 lb. lean ground beef
½ cup chopped onion
¾ cup chunky salsa
2 cups shredded Colby-Jack cheese
10–12 flour tortillas

Brown ground beef with onion. Drain. Mix in salsa and cheese. If freezing, see directions below. Otherwise, spoon approximately ½ cup of meat mixture on one half of tortilla. Fold tortilla in half to close. Arrange quesadillas on baking sheet. Lightly spray tops of tortillas with cooking spray. Bake at 450° for 8 minutes or until lightly browned.

Freezing directions: Place meat mixture in a freezer bag. Include a package of flour tortillas with this meal.

Beef Stroganoff

The longer you cook this, the more tender the meat becomes.

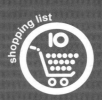

⅓ cup flour
2 cups milk
2 tsp. beef bouillon granules
1–1½ lbs. lean stew meat
½ packet dry onion soup mix
1 bay leaf
1 small can sliced mushrooms
½ cup water
2 cups sour cream
1 small pkg. egg noodles

To make a white sauce with the first 3 ingredients, warm about 1½ cups of the milk in a saucepan. Place all the flour and beef granules in a mixing bowl and gradually whisk in the remaining milk until no lumps remain. Slowly add it to the warm milk in the saucepan. Stirring constantly over medium heat, bring the sauce to a gentle boil. Allow to boil for 1 minute, stirring constantly. Remove saucepan from heat. Add the rest of the ingredients to the sauce except for the sour cream. If freezing, see directions below. Otherwise, pour in a slow cooker and cook for 6 hours on low until meat is tender. Add sour cream just before serving. Serve over noodles.

shopping list

- 3⅓ cups flour
- 20 cups milk
- Abt. ½ cup beef bouillon granules
- 10–15 lbs. lean stew meat
- 5 packets dry onion soup mix
- 10 bay leaves
- 10 small cans sliced mushrooms
- 10 pints sour cream
- 10 pkgs. noodles

Freezing directions: Cool and place in a freezer bag. Include a pint of sour cream and a package of noodles with each meal. (Do not freeze sour cream.)

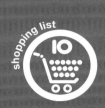

- 20 lbs. ground beef
- ¼ cup salt
- 2 Tbsp. pepper
- 5 onions
- 30 eggs
- 20 potatoes
- 40 carrots
- 7½ cups milk
- 20 cans cream of chicken soup
- 20 cans cream of mushroom soup
- 10 cans evaporated milk
- 10 pkgs. rice or noodles

Creamy Meatballs

If you are short on time, you can buy the meatballs,
but this is a terrific, hearty meatball recipe.

2 lbs. ground beef
2 tsp. salt
1 tsp. pepper
½ onion, grated
3 eggs
2 potatoes, grated
4 carrots, grated
¾ cup milk

Sauce:
2 cans cream of chicken soup
2 cans cream of mushroom soup
1 can evaporated milk

Combine meatball ingredients and form into balls. Place on a cookie sheet and bake at 400° for 20 minutes. Mix sauce; add cooked meatballs. If freezing, see directions below. Otherwise, place in a 9×13 casserole dish and bake at 350° for 30–45 minutes or until bubbly. Serve over rice or noodles.

Freezing directions: Pour sauce over cooked meatballs in a freezer bag. You may want to include a package of rice or noodles with this meal.

Easy Swedish Meatballs

It doesn't get any easier than these!

30 pre-cooked frozen meatballs
1 pkg. country gravy mix
1 cup sour cream
1 (12 oz.) pkg. egg noodles

Prepare gravy according to package directions. In a large saucepan, mix prepared gravy with 1 cup sour cream. If freezing, see directions below. Otherwise, add frozen meatballs. Heat until meatballs are cooked through and the mixture is bubbly. Serve over prepared noodles.

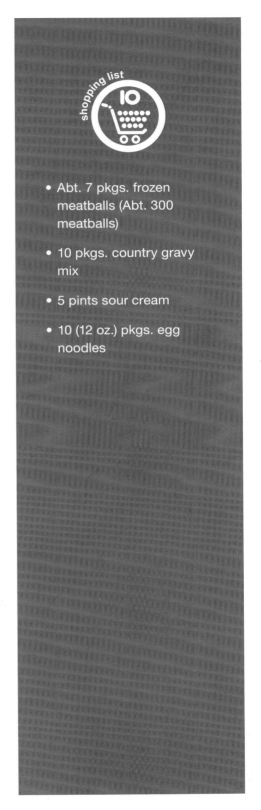

shopping list

- Abt. 7 pkgs. frozen meatballs (Abt. 300 meatballs)

- 10 pkgs. country gravy mix

- 5 pints sour cream

- 10 (12 oz.) pkgs. egg noodles

Freezing directions: Mix prepared gravy with sour cream. Place meatballs in a freezer bag and pour sauce over the meatballs.

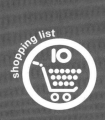
- 10 lbs. ground beef

- 10 cups Italian bread crumbs

- 5 cups shredded parmesan cheese

- Abt. ⅔ cup fresh minced parsley or 3½ Tbsp. dried

- 1 bulb of garlic

- 5 cups milk

- 10 eggs

- 20 (15 oz.) cans tomato sauce

- 10 (29 oz.) can crushed Italian tomatoes

- 20 spaghetti sauce seasoning envelopes

- 10 pkgs. hogi buns

- 4 lbs. shredded mozzarella or provolone cheese

Italian Meatball Subs

The spaghetti sauce seasoning thickens the sauce perfectly and adds the right balance of flavor.

Meatball ingredients:
   1 lb. lean ground beef
   1 cup Italian bread crumbs
   ½ cup shredded parmesan cheese
   1 Tbsp. fresh minced parsley (or 1 tsp. dried)
   1 garlic clove, minced
   ½ cup milk
   1 egg

Sauce ingredients:
   2 (15 oz.) can tomato sauce
   1 (29 oz.) can crushed Italian tomatoes
   ½ cup shredded parmesan cheese
   2 envelopes spaghetti sauce seasoning

To serve:
   hogi buns
   shredded mozzarella or provolone cheese

Combine meatball ingredients in a large bowl. Set aside. In another large bowl, combine the sauce ingredients and stir until well mixed. Pour about ⅓ of the sauce mixture in the bottom of a large slow cooker. Form the meatballs from the meat mixture and put them in a single layer in the sauce in the slow cooker. Add some sauce to cover the tops and sides of the meatballs. Add more meatballs and cover with more sauce. When all the meatballs are in the slow cooker, pour the rest of the sauce on and cover. Cook on low for 8 hours or high for 4 hours.

Freezing directions: After cooking, allow to cool. Pour into freezer bags. To serve, heat in a large saucepan. Serve on buns with shredded cheese on top. Include a bag of 1½ cups of shredded cheese and a package of buns.

Meatloaf

To cut down on the fat content, use extra-lean ground beef and turkey bacon.

2 lbs. ground beef
1 envelope beefy mushroom soup mix
¾ cup saltine crackers
2 eggs
¾ cup water
⅓ cup ketchup
¼ tsp. seasoned salt
⅛ tsp. garlic salt
¼ cup chopped green pepper (optional)
¼ cup chopped onion (optional)
6 strips bacon

Combine all ingredients except the bacon. Place in a large loaf pan or 2 smaller pans. Cover with strips of bacon. If freezing, see directions below. Otherwise, bake at 350° for 1 hour until done. Let stand for 10 minutes before slicing.

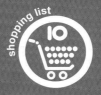

- 20 lbs. ground beef

- 10 envelopes beefy mushroom soup mix

- Abt. 1½ boxes saltine crackers (6 sleeves)

- 20 eggs

- 3⅓ cups ketchup

- 2½ tsp. seasoned salt

- 1½ tsp. garlic salt

- 3 large green peppers

- 3 large onions

- Abt. 5 pkgs. bacon (60 slices)

Freezing directions: Place it in 2 disposable aluminum loaf pans, or shape it into a large loaf and place it in a 9×13 pan. To freeze, wrap loaf in foil or place in a freezer bag to prevent freezer burn.

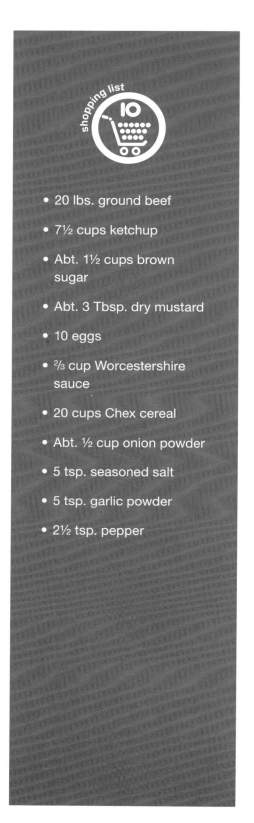

- 20 lbs. ground beef
- 7½ cups ketchup
- Abt. 1½ cups brown sugar
- Abt. 3 Tbsp. dry mustard
- 10 eggs
- ⅔ cup Worcestershire sauce
- 20 cups Chex cereal
- Abt. ½ cup onion powder
- 5 tsp. seasoned salt
- 5 tsp. garlic powder
- 2½ tsp. pepper

Mini Meatloaves

Meatloaf is so easy to prepare in large quantities!

¾ cup ketchup
2–3 Tbsp. brown sugar
¾ tsp. dry mustard
1 egg, beaten
3 tsp. Worcestershire sauce
2 cups Chex cereal, crushed
2 tsp. onion powder
½ tsp. seasoned salt
½ tsp. garlic powder
¼ tsp. pepper
2 lbs. ground beef

In a large bowl, combine ketchup, brown sugar, and dry mustard. Set aside ⅓ cup of this mixture for the topping. Add egg, Worcestershire sauce, crushed cereal, onion powder, seasoned salt, garlic powder, and pepper to mixture. Crumble in ground beef and mix all together. Press meat mixture into 12 muffin cups (about ⅓ cup each). If freezing, see directions below. Otherwise, bake at 375° for 20–25 minutes. Spoon remaining ketchup mixture on top and bake 10 minutes longer or until meat is no longer pink.

Freezing directions: Flash freeze Meatloaves in muffin tins. Remove from pan and place in a gallon-size freezer bag. Seal and freeze. These can be baked on a baking sheet after they are thawed. Include topping in a quart-size freezer bag.

Navajo Tacos

This is a fun variation of regular tacos!

12 Rhodes Texas rolls, thawed and risen
vegetable oil for frying
1 lb. ground beef
1 (15 oz.) can pinto beans
1 envelope taco seasoning
2 cups shredded cheddar cheese
2 cups shredded lettuce
2 medium tomatoes, diced
1 medium onion, chopped
1 cup sour cream
1 cup salsa

Flatten each roll to a 6-inch circle. Fry each side in vegetable oil at 375° until golden brown. Follow directions on taco seasoning package to prepare ground beef. Add pinto beans and heat through. If freezing, see directions below. Otherwise, place desired amount of ground beef mixture on warm fry bread. Top with desired toppings.

 Freezing directions: Place frozen rolls in quantities of 8–10 in a freezer bag. Prepare meat as directed; allow to cool and place in a freezer bag. Include a bag of cheese with the freezer items along with the fresh produce and a carton of sour cream to refrigerate and use within a week. (Do not freeze sour cream.) Have group members use their own salsa.

shopping list

- 5 bags Rhodes Texas rolls (24 rolls per bag)

- 10 lbs. ground beef

- 10 (15 oz.) cans pinto beans

- 10 envelopes taco seasoning

- 5 lbs. shredded cheddar cheese

- Abt. 5 heads lettuce (or divided bags of shredded lettuce to save time)

- 20 medium tomatoes

- 10 medium onions

- 10 small containers sour cream

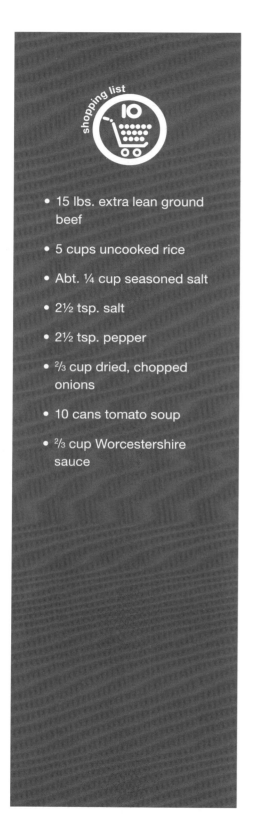

- 15 lbs. extra lean ground beef

- 5 cups uncooked rice

- Abt. ¼ cup seasoned salt

- 2½ tsp. salt

- 2½ tsp. pepper

- ⅔ cup dried, chopped onions

- 10 cans tomato soup

- ⅔ cup Worcestershire sauce

Porcupine Meatballs

You would need a porcupine to keep your kids away from these meatballs!

1½ lbs. extra lean ground beef
½ cup uncooked rice
1 tsp. seasoned salt
¼ tsp. salt
½ tsp. pepper
1 Tbsp. dried, chopped onions
1 can tomato soup
1 Tbsp. Worcestershire sauce

Combine ground beef, rice, salts, pepper, and onions. Mix well. Place in a 9×13 pan. Mix together Worcestershire sauce and tomato soup and pour over meatballs. If freezing, see directions below. Otherwise, cover and bake at 350° for 1–1½ hours until rice is tender. Turn meatballs halfway through baking.

Freezing directions: Place in a disposable aluminum pan. Cover with foil.

Salisbury Steaks

Pair these up with rice, a green salad, and rolls, and you have a simple Sunday meal.

2 lbs. ground beef (for best results, use the leanest ground beef you can find)
½ cup crushed saltine crackers
2 eggs, slightly beaten
¼ cup milk
1 Tbsp. Savory Herb with Garlic soup mix
2 envelopes beef or mushroom gravy mix

Combine ground beef, cracker crumbs, eggs, milk, and soup mix. Mix thoroughly. Shape into patties (6–8). If freezing, see directions below. Otherwise, follow desired cooking directions.

Skillet method: Brown patties in a skillet. Mix gravy according to package directions, pour over patties, and simmer until done.

Slow cooker method: Put patties in a slow cooker. Mix gravy according to package directions and pour over patties. Cook on medium for 4–6 hours.

Freezing directions: Place wax paper between each patty or flash freeze. Place in a freezer bag. Include 2 packages of gravy mix with each meal.

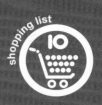

- 20 lbs. ground beef (extra lean)

- 1 box saltine crackers

- 20 eggs

- 2½ cups milk

- 1 box (3 pkgs.) Savory Herb with Garlic soup mix

- 20 envelopes beef or mushroom gravy mix

shopping list

- 10 rump roasts

- 20 envelopes au jus mix

- 10 pkgs. rolls

Shredded Beef French Dip Sandwiches

Serve this with chips and carrot sticks to make your meal finger-friendly.

1 rump roast
2 envelopes au jus mix
1 pkg. rolls (6–8 deli rolls or 12–18 hard rolls)

Place roast beef in slow cooker and cook on medium for 3–6 hours until it shreds easily. Halfway through cooking, take the roast out, cut off the fat, and drain juices. Place back in slow cooker. Prepare au jus according to package directions and pour over roast. Cook for the remaining amount of time until it shreds. If freezing, see directions below. Otherwise, serve on rolls and dip in au jus.

Freezing directions: Place meat and prepared au jus in a freezer bag. Include a bag of rolls with this meal. To prepare this meal in bulk, you can place approximately 5 roasts in a large roaster oven.

Sloppy Joes

Filling and hearty—we love these with tater tots and a fruit salad. Yummy, yummy!

1½ lbs. ground beef, browned
1 chopped onion
¼ tsp. garlic powder
1 (12 oz.) jar chili sauce
½ cup brown sugar
2 Tbsp. vinegar
2 Tbsp. prepared mustard
1 (16 oz.) can tomato sauce
1 pkg. hamburger buns

Mix all ingredients together. Simmer for 15–20 minutes. If freezing, see directions below. Otherwise, serve on hamburger buns.

- 15 lbs. ground beef

- 10 onions

- 2½ tsp. garlic powder

- 10 (12 oz.) jars chili sauce

- 5 cups brown sugar

- 1¼ cup vinegar

- 1¼ cup prepared mustard

- 10 (16 oz.) cans tomato sauce

- 10 pkgs. hamburger buns

- 10 pkgs. potato chips (optional)

Freezing directions: Freeze in a gallon-size freezer bag. Include a package of hamburger buns (freeze in a freezer bag as well). You might want to include a bag of potato chips with this meal.

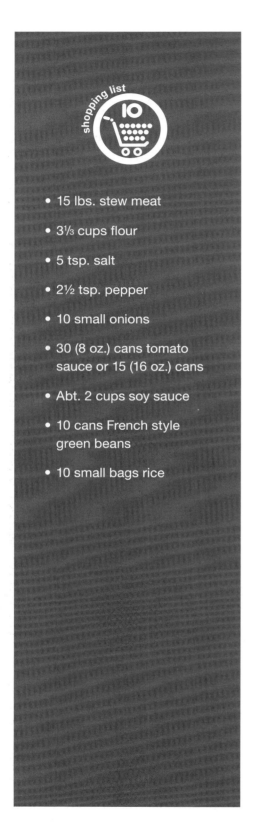

shopping list
10

- 15 lbs. stew meat

- 3⅓ cups flour

- 5 tsp. salt

- 2½ tsp. pepper

- 10 small onions

- 30 (8 oz.) cans tomato sauce or 15 (16 oz.) cans

- Abt. 2 cups soy sauce

- 10 cans French style green beans

- 10 small bags rice

Smothered Steak

This saucy dish is a real treat after a long day's work.

1½ lbs. stew meat
⅓ cup flour
½ tsp. salt
¼ tsp. pepper
1 small chopped onion
3 (8 oz.) cans tomato sauce
3 Tbsp. soy sauce
1 can French style green beans

If freezing, see directions below. Otherwise, put steak, flour, salt, and pepper in a slow cooker. Stir well to coat meat. Add all remaining ingredients. Cover and cook 6–8 hours. Serve over rice.

Freezing directions: Place flour, salt, and pepper in a freezer bag. Place meat in the bag and shake to coat. Mix all remaining ingredients except green beans together and pour over meat. Freeze flat in freezer. Include the can of green beans with the meal. Mix the beans in the slow cooker with the other ingredients to cook. You may want to include a bag of rice with this meal.

Stuffed Green Peppers

The meat mixture is also great just in the muffin tins without the green peppers for small ones who may not like the peppers.

1 lb. ground beef, browned and drained
⅓ cup minced onions
½ tsp. salt
½ tsp. pepper
3 (8 oz.) cans tomato sauce
¾ cup water
½ cup uncooked long grain rice
1 tsp. Worcestershire sauce
1 cup shredded cheddar cheese
6 medium green peppers with tops off and seeds cleaned out

Mix all ingredients except cheese and green peppers together. Cover and simmer 15–20 minutes until rice is tender. Stir in cheese. Spoon mixture into green peppers. If freezing, see directions below. Otherwise, place in muffin tins and bake at 350° for 30–35 minutes.

Freezing directions: After spooning the meat mixture into the peppers, wrap peppers in foil and place in a freezer bag to freeze. You can also freeze the meat and the peppers separately.

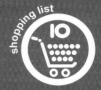

shopping list

- 10 lbs. ground beef
- 4 large onions
- 5 tsp. salt
- 5 tsp. pepper
- 30 (8 oz.) cans tomato sauce or 15 (16 oz.) cans
- 5 cups long grain rice
- 10 tsp. Worcestershire sauce
- 2½ lbs. shredded cheddar cheese
- 60 green peppers

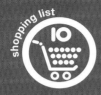
- 10 lbs. ground beef

- 5 cups dry bread crumbs

- 2½ cups milk

- 2½ Tbsp. salt

- 5 tsp. Worcestershire sauce

- 2½ tsp. pepper

- 3 large onions

- 10 eggs

- 5 cups brown sugar

- Abt. ¼ cup powdered mustard

- 5 tsp. nutmeg

- Abt. 4 (24 oz.) bottles ketchup (total of 80 oz.)

Sweet and Sour Meatballs

This is a welcome change from your typical sweet and sour recipes.

1 lb. ground beef
½ cup dry bread crumbs
¼ cup milk
¾ tsp. salt
½ tsp. Worcestershire sauce
¼ tsp. pepper
¼ cup onion, minced
1 egg

Mix all together and form balls. Bake on a cookie sheet at 400° for 20 minutes.

Sauce:
½ cup brown sugar
2 tsp. dry mustard
½ tsp. nutmeg
1 cup ketchup

Mix sauce ingredients together. If freezing, see directions below. Otherwise, place meatballs in a slow cooker and pour sauce over them. Mix to coat meatballs and cook on low for 2–3 hours.

Freezing directions: Place meatballs in a freezer bag and pour sauce over them.

Taco Braid

A new twist on taco night!

1 lb. ground beef, browned and drained
1 pkg. taco seasoning
12 Rhodes rolls, thawed
1 (15 oz.) can refried beans
2 cups shredded cheddar cheese

Follow directions on taco seasoning packet to season ground beef. Roll out rolls together into a rectangle about the length of a cookie sheet. Spread refried beans down the center of the dough. Top with meat mixture and then sprinkle with the shredded cheese. Use a pizza cutter to cut strips along each side of the dough (even numbers on each side). Starting at the bottom, take each piece, cross, and twist. Crisscross dough across top of filling. Continue crisscrossing until your pizza is braided. Carefully place on a greased cookie sheet. If freezing, see directions below. Otherwise, place on a cookie sheet and bake at 350° for 25–30 minutes until bread is golden brown.

Freezing directions: Wrap braid with plastic wrap and then aluminum foil. Freeze.

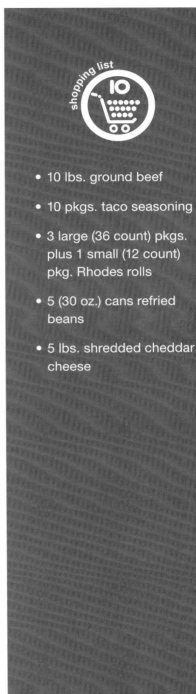

shopping list

- 10 lbs. ground beef

- 10 pkgs. taco seasoning

- 3 large (36 count) pkgs. plus 1 small (12 count) pkg. Rhodes rolls

- 5 (30 oz.) cans refried beans

- 5 lbs. shredded cheddar cheese

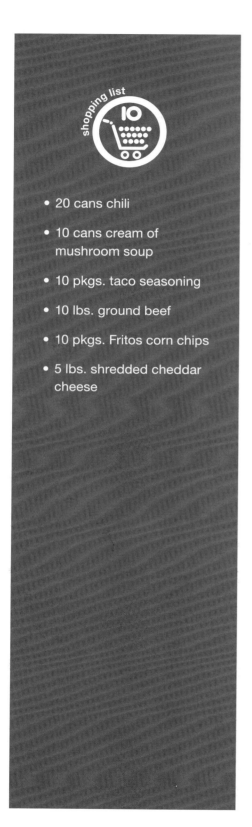

shopping list

10

- 20 cans chili

- 10 cans cream of mushroom soup

- 10 pkgs. taco seasoning

- 10 lbs. ground beef

- 10 pkgs. Fritos corn chips

- 5 lbs. shredded cheddar cheese

Taco Casserole

Another simple but fun Mexican-themed dish.

2 (15 oz.) cans chili
1 can cream of mushroom soup
1 pkg. taco seasoning
1 lb. ground beef, browned and drained
1 pkg. Fritos corn chips
2 cups shredded cheddar cheese, divided

Mix together chili, soup, taco seasoning, 1 cup of cheese, and ground beef. If freezing, see directions below. Otherwise, place the meat mixture in a 9×13 pan and top with chips. Bake at 350° for 30 minutes or until bubbly. Take out of oven and top with remaining cheese. Top with other family favorites such as sour cream, olives, tomatoes, and salsa.

Freezing directions: Place meat mixture in a gallon-size freezer bag; seal and freeze. Include a bag of Fritos and 1 cup shredded cheese.

Tamale Pie

This not-too-spicy pie goes over well with little ones
who have sensitive taste buds.

1 lb. ground beef, browned
1 (15 oz.) can corn, drained
1 small can sliced olives
1 clove minced garlic
1 Tbsp. sugar
1 tsp. salt
1 Tbsp. chili powder
1 (15 oz.) can beans (white, kidney, or pinto), drained
1½ cups shredded cheese
2 (8 oz.) cans tomato sauce

Combine all ingredients and place in a 9×13 baking dish.

To make crust, combine the following in a saucepan on medium to high heat:

1 cup cornmeal
2½ cups cold water
1½ tsp. salt

Stir frequently until thick. Add 1 tablespoon butter and stir until melted.
Spread crust mixture on top of meat mixture. If freezing, see directions below.
Otherwise, cover and bake at 375° for 40 minutes.

Freezing directions: Place in a disposable aluminum pan. Cover
tightly and freeze.

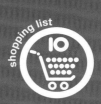

- 10 lbs. ground beef

- 10 (15 oz.) cans corn

- 10 small can sliced olives

- 2 bunches garlic

- Abt. ⅔ cup sugar

- Abt. ½ cup salt

- Abt. ⅔ cup chili powder

- 10 cans beans

- 20 (8 oz.) cans tomato sauce

- 4 lbs. shredded cheese

- 10 cups cornmeal

- ½ cup plus 2 Tbsp. butter

Chicken Recipes

- See page 16 for ideas on cooking chicken in bulk.

- If it is a slow cooker meal, freeze in a bag.

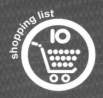

- 30 lbs. boneless skinless chicken breasts
- 10 cups ketchup
- 10 cups vinegar
- 5 cups molasses
- 5 cups honey
- Abt. ¼ cup liquid smoke
- 5 tsp. salt
- 2½ tsp. garlic powder
- 2½ tsp. onion powder
- 2½ tsp. hot sauce (Tabasco)
- 10 pkgs. buns

Barbecue Chicken Sandwiches

Your favorite barbecue restaurant doesn't even compare to the tangy barbecue sauce in these sandwiches!

1 cup ketchup
1 cup vinegar
½ cup molasses
½ cup honey
1 tsp. liquid smoke
½ tsp. salt
¼ tsp. garlic powder
¼ tsp. onion powder
¼ tsp. hot sauce (Tabasco; optional)
2–3 lbs. boneless, skinless chicken breasts

Combine all ingredients except chicken in a saucepan over high heat. Blend with a whisk until smooth. When the mixture comes to a boil, add the chicken. Turn the heat down and simmer for 45–60 minutes. Once the chicken is tender enough to shred and the sauce is thickened, remove from heat and shred the chicken with two forks. If freezing, see directions below. Otherwise, serve on buns.

Freezing directions: After shredding the chicken, allow to cool. Pour into a freezer bag. You can also cook this in a slow cooker.

Breaded Ranch Chicken

This chicken will have your mouth watering for more.

6 boneless, skinless chicken breasts
1 cup ranch dressing
1 cup Italian style bread crumbs
3 Tbsp. minced onions
1 lb. cooked and crumbled bacon (or 1 cup pre-cooked bacon pieces)

Mix bread crumbs, onions, and bacon together. Dip chicken in ranch and then cover with bread crumb mixture. If freezing, see directions below. Otherwise, place in a 9×13 pan and bake at 375° for 1 hour.

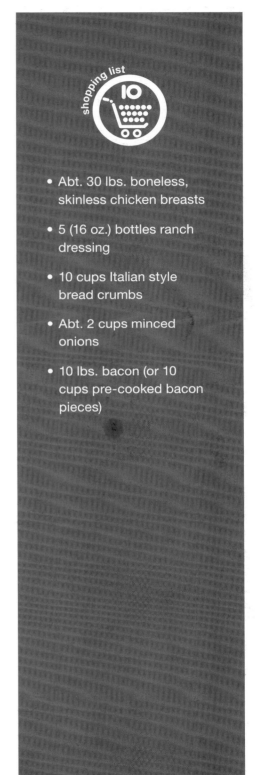

shopping list

- Abt. 30 lbs. boneless, skinless chicken breasts

- 5 (16 oz.) bottles ranch dressing

- 10 cups Italian style bread crumbs

- Abt. 2 cups minced onions

- 10 lbs. bacon (or 10 cups pre-cooked bacon pieces)

Freezing directions: Place in a disposable aluminum pan; cover with foil and freeze.

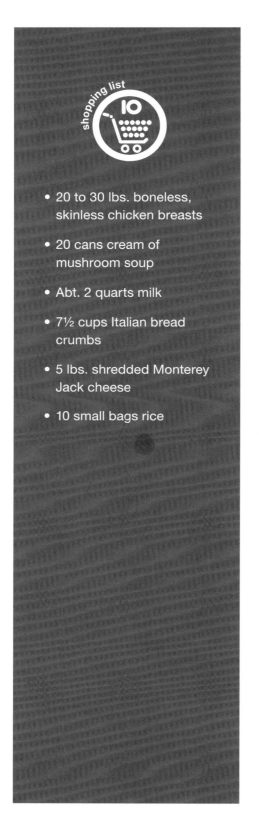

shopping list

- 20 to 30 lbs. boneless, skinless chicken breasts

- 20 cans cream of mushroom soup

- Abt. 2 quarts milk

- 7½ cups Italian bread crumbs

- 5 lbs. shredded Monterey Jack cheese

- 10 small bags rice

Cheesy Italian Chicken

Easy and cheesy—this is a dish that gets repeat requests!

4–6 boneless, skinless chicken breasts, cut in pieces
2 cans cream of chicken soup
¾ cup milk
¾ cup Italian bread crumbs
2 cups Monterey Jack cheese

Mix soup, milk, bread crumbs, and cheese together. Add chicken pieces. If freezing, see directions below. Otherwise, cook in slow cooker on low for 6–8 hours. Stir often so cheese doesn't stick to the bottom. Serve over rice or noodles.

Freezing directions: Place chicken pieces in a freezer bag. Mix all other ingredients together and pour over chicken in the bag. You may want to include a bag of rice with this meal.

Chicken Broccoli Rice Bake

Comfort food at its best!

4 chicken breasts (cooked and cut up)
1 pkg. chicken-flavored rice mix (prepared according to pkg. directions)
2 Tbsp. butter or margarine (to prepare rice)
1 (16 oz.) pkg. frozen broccoli
2–3 cups shredded cheddar cheese
1 sleeve crushed saltine crackers
2 Tbsp. butter or margarine

Sauce:
2 cans cream of chicken soup
1 cup mayonnaise
2 tsp. lemon juice
1 Tbsp. curry powder (optional)
¼ cup milk

Spread prepared rice in the bottom of a 9×13 baking dish. Mix sauce ingredients together. Spread ⅓ of the sauce over rice. Layer the broccoli and spread ⅓ of the sauce on top. Evenly spread chicken on top of the sauce and add remaining sauce on top. Top with cheese. If freezing, see directions below. Otherwise, top with crushed crackers and dabs of butter (butter optional). Bake at 375° for 45–55 minutes.

Freezing directions: Slightly undercook rice to freeze. Place meal in a disposable aluminum pan; cover and freeze. Before baking, top with crushed crackers and dabs of butter (butter optional). Include butter and crackers along with this meal.

shopping list

- 20 lbs. chicken breasts
- 10 pkgs. chicken flavored rice mix
- 10 pkgs. frozen broccoli
- 6 lbs. shredded cheddar cheese
- 3 pkgs. saltine crackers (with 4 sleeves each)
- 2½ cups butter or margarine
- 20 cans cream of chicken soup
- 3 (32 oz.) jars mayonnaise
- Abt. ¼ cup lemon juice
- ⅔ cup curry powder (optional)
- 2½ cups milk

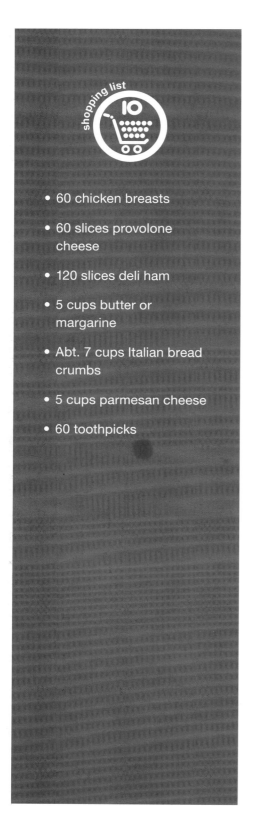

shopping list 10

- 60 chicken breasts
- 60 slices provolone cheese
- 120 slices deli ham
- 5 cups butter or margarine
- Abt. 7 cups Italian bread crumbs
- 5 cups parmesan cheese
- 60 toothpicks

Chicken Cordon Bleu

Who doesn't love the combined flavors of chicken, cheese, and ham?

6 chicken breasts
6 slices provolone cheese
12 slices deli ham
½ cup butter or margarine, melted
⅔ cups Italian bread crumbs
½ cup parmesan cheese

Pound chicken breasts until they are ½ inch thick. In a medium sized bowl, mix bread crumbs and parmesan cheese. Put 2 slices of ham on the chicken. Roll up a slice of provolone cheese and place in the center of meat. Roll up meat and secure with a toothpick. Dip in melted butter and then in bread crumb mixture. If freezing, see directions below. Otherwise, place seam-side down on cookie sheet. Cover and bake at 350° for 30 minutes or until chicken is no longer pink.

Optional: You can also use turkey tenders for this recipe.

Freezing directions: Place in a freezer bag and freeze.

Chicken Divan

Leave the curry out if there are sensitive taste buds in your home. However, it does add a nice kick!

6 boneless skinless chicken breasts, cooked and diced
2 (10 oz.) pkgs. chopped broccoli
1 cup mayonnaise
2 cans cream of chicken soup
1 tsp. lemon juice
1 tsp. curry powder
1 cup shredded cheddar cheese
½ cup dry bread crumbs
2 Tbsp. melted butter

Cook broccoli as directed on package. Drain. Mix all ingredients except cheese and bread crumbs. Include cheese and bread crumbs with this meal. If freezing, see directions below. Otherwise, place in a 9×13 casserole dish. Cover with cheese. Mix the bread crumbs with the melted butter and sprinkle on top. Bake at 350° for 25 minutes. Serve over cooked rice.

Freezing directions: Slightly undercook broccoli. Place in a disposable aluminum pan and cover tightly with foil.

shopping list

- 60 boneless, skinless chicken breasts
- 20 (10 oz.) pkgs. chopped broccoli
- 10 cups mayonnaise
- 20 cans cream of chicken soup
- Abt. ½ cup lemon juice
- Abt. ½ cup curry powder
- 10 cups shredded cheddar cheese
- 5 cups bread crumbs
- 1¼ cup butter

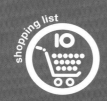
- Abt. 1 cup yeast

- Abt. 2 cups sugar

- ¾ cup salt

- 3⅓ cups oil

- 60 cups flour

- 10 pkgs. cream cheese

- 5 cubes butter

- 2½ cups milk

- 2½ tsp. pepper

- 15 cups Italian bread crumbs

- 2 bunches green onions

- 10 cans cream of chicken soup

- 12 lbs. boneless, skinless chicken breasts

Chicken Pockets

To save time, you can use refrigerator crescent rolls, but the homemade dough is well worth the effort.

Dough (2 hour French bread dough):
    ½ cup warm water
    1 Tbsp. plus 1 tsp. yeast
    3 Tbsp. sugar
    1 Tbsp. salt
    ⅓ cup oil
    2 cups very hot tap water
    6 cups flour

Chicken Pockets:
    1 batch of 2-hour French bread dough
    8 oz. cream cheese
    4 Tbsp. melted butter
    ½ tsp. salt
    ¼ tsp. pepper
    2 Tbsp. chopped green onions
    2 cups cooked and cubed chicken
    4 Tbsp. milk
    1½ cups Italian bread crumbs

Chicken gravy:
    1 can cream of chicken soup
    ¾ cup water or milk

Dissolve yeast and sugar in ½ cup water. In a large bowl, combine salt, oil, and 2 cups hot water. Mix in 3 cups flour. Add the yeast mixture. Mix in remaining 3 cups of flour. Punch down every 10 minutes for 50 minutes. If making Chicken Pockets, continue on to the next part of the recipe. If making French bread, shape, and let rise until double. Bake at 400° for 20 minutes. (Also great for sweet rolls.)

Blend cream cheese and melted butter until smooth. Add the remaining ingredients. Roll out bread dough and cut into 3-inch squares. Place ½ cup of chicken mixture in the center of each square. Pull up the corners and seal the edges. Roll in melted butter and then in bread crumbs. Let rise until double in size. If freezing, see directions below. Otherwise, bake at 350° for 20 minutes or until golden brown. Serve with chicken gravy.

Empty can of soup into saucepan and whisk in water or milk. Heat until very warm, stirring continually. Serve over chicken pockets.

Freezing directions: Flash freeze chicken pockets and place in a freezer bag. Include a can of cream of chicken soup with each meal for group members to prepare the gravy at home.

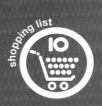

- Abt. 20 lbs. boneless, skinless chicken breasts

- 15 cups elbow macaroni

- 5 lbs. shredded cheddar cheese

- 10 cans cream of chicken soup

- 2½ quarts milk

- 10 (8 oz.) cans mushrooms (optional)

- 2½ tsp. pepper

Chicken Macaroni Bake

Homemade macaroni and cheese taste with less work.

2 cups chicken, cooked and cubed
1½ cups uncooked elbow macaroni
2 cups shredded cheddar cheese
1 can cream of chicken soup
1 cup milk
1 (8 oz.) can mushrooms (optional), drained
¼ tsp. pepper

In a large bowl, combine the chicken, macaroni, cheese, soup, milk, mushrooms, and pepper. If freezing, see directions below. Otherwise, pour into a greased 9×13 pan. Cover and bake at 350° for 60–65 minutes or until macaroni is tender.

Freezing directions: May freeze in a freezer bag or a disposable aluminum pan.

Chicken Marango

The combination of these ingredients makes a great, flavorful chicken.

6 boneless, skinless chicken breasts
1 can tomato soup
1 can Golden Mushroom soup
1 can mushrooms, drained
½ cup chopped onion

Mix soups, mushrooms and onion. If freezing, see directions below. Otherwise, pour mixture over chicken in slow cooker and cook on low for 6–8 hours. Serve over warm noodles.

Freezing directions: Place chicken in freezer bag. Pour mixture over chicken and seal. Include a package of noodles with this meal.

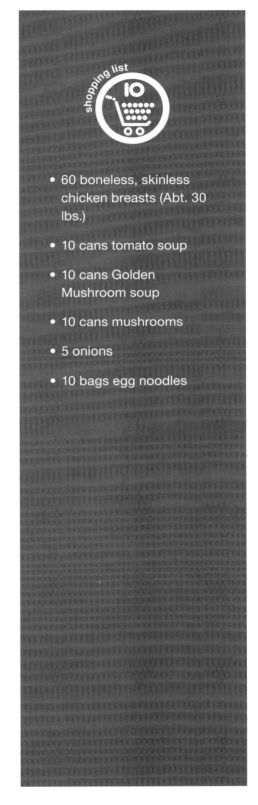

shopping list

- 60 boneless, skinless chicken breasts (Abt. 30 lbs.)
- 10 cans tomato soup
- 10 cans Golden Mushroom soup
- 10 cans mushrooms
- 5 onions
- 10 bags egg noodles

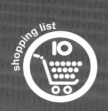

shopping list 10

- 10 (16 oz.) pkgs. of noodles

- 5 cups mayonnaise

- 5 cups milk

- 10 cans cream of chicken soup

- 10 large cans chicken

- 10 cups shredded cheddar cheese

- Abt. 3 Tbsp. garlic salt

- Abt. 3 Tbsp. seasoned salt

- Abt. 2 Tbsp. pepper

- 10 small cans French's onions

Chicken Noodle Casserole

You can never have too many great chicken recipes.

1 (16 oz.) pkg. wide egg noodles
½ cup mayonnaise
½ cup milk
1 can cream of chicken soup
1 large can chicken (drained)
2 cups shredded cheddar cheese (divided)
garlic salt to taste
seasoned salt to taste
dash of pepper
1 small can French's onions

Cook noodles according to package directions. In a large mixing bowl, mix together mayonnaise, milk, soup, and chicken. Season to taste. Drain the pasta; stir into chicken mixture. Then stir in 1 cup of cheese. Add the remaining cup of cheese on top and top with onions. If freezing, see directions below. Otherwise, bake at 425° for 20–25 minutes until bubbly.

Freezing directions: When preparing, undercook the noodles. Put in a disposable aluminum pan and cover tightly with foil. If you bake this one from frozen, keep it covered for the first half of baking.

Chicken Tetrazzini

You can also use leftover turkey in this terrific recipe.

8 oz. spaghetti, broken in pieces
5 Tbsp. butter or margarine
6 Tbsp. flour
3 cups chicken broth
1 cup light cream
1 tsp. salt
dash of pepper
1 small can mushrooms, undrained
5 Tbsp. minced green peppers
3 cups cooked chicken, cubed
½ cup shredded parmesan cheese
1 cup shredded cheddar cheese

Cook spaghetti according to package directions. In a medium saucepan, melt butter and blend in flour. Stir broth into mixture and add cream. Cook until mixture thickens and bubbles, stirring constantly. Add salt, pepper, drained spaghetti, mushrooms, green peppers, and cooked chicken. Place in a 9×13 pan and sprinkle with parmesan and cheddar cheese. If freezing, see directions below. Otherwise, bake at 350° for 30–45 minutes until bubbly and lightly browned.

 Freezing directions: Slightly undercook spaghetti. Place in a disposable aluminum pan; cover and freeze.

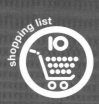

shopping list

- 10 (8 oz.) pkgs. spaghetti
- 3¼ cups butter or margarine
- 3¾ cups flour
- 30 cups chicken broth
- 5 pints light cream
- Abt. ¼ cup salt
- Abt. 2 Tbsp. pepper
- 10 small cans mushrooms
- 5 green peppers
- 15 lbs. boneless skinless chicken breasts
- 5 cups parmesan cheese
- 2½ lbs. shredded cheddar cheese

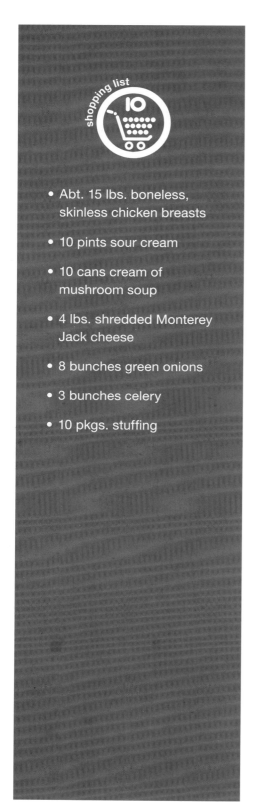

shopping list
10

- Abt. 15 lbs. boneless, skinless chicken breasts

- 10 pints sour cream

- 10 cans cream of mushroom soup

- 4 lbs. shredded Monterey Jack cheese

- 8 bunches green onions

- 3 bunches celery

- 10 pkgs. stuffing

Company's Coming Chicken

Don't save this one for company—it's too good!

2½ cups chicken, cooked and cubed
2 cups sour cream
1 can cream of mushroom soup
1½ cups Monterey Jack cheese, shredded
½ cup green onions
½ cup chopped celery
1 pkg. stuffing, prepared

Place chicken in a 9×13 pan. Combine sour cream, soup, cheese, green onions, and celery. Spoon mixture over chicken. Prepare stuffing and sprinkle over mixture. If freezing, see directions below. Otherwise, bake at 375° for 35 to 40 minutes.

Freezing directions: Place in a disposable aluminum pan and cover tightly with foil to freeze.

Creamy Bacon Chicken

Rich and creamy!

5–6 boneless, skinless chicken breasts
1 (3 oz.) pkg. precooked bacon bits (not artificial)
1 can roasted garlic cream of mushroom soup
1 can cream of mushroom soup
1 cup sour cream
½ cup flour

If freezing, see directions below. Otherwise, place chicken in slow cooker. Mix all remaining ingredients together and pour over chicken. Cook on low for 6–8 hours. Serve over egg noodles.

Freezing directions: Place chicken in a gallon-size freezer bag. Pour sauce mixture over chicken. Seal and freeze. You may want to include a bag of egg noodles with this meal.

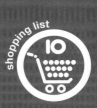

shopping list

- Abt. 30 lbs. boneless, skinless chicken breasts

- 10 (3 oz.) pkgs. precooked bacon bits (not artificial)

- 10 cans roasted garlic cream of mushroom soup

- 10 cans cream of mushroom soup

- 5 pints sour cream

- 5 cups flour

- 10 pkgs. egg noodles

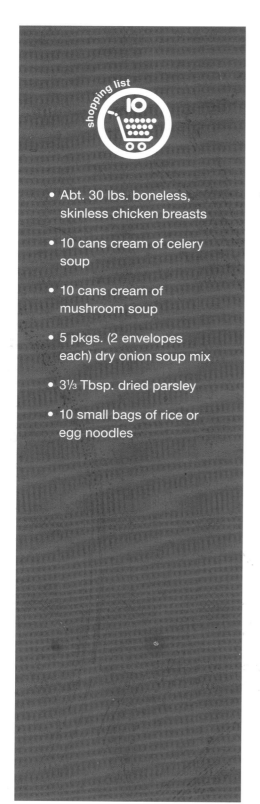

shopping list 10

- Abt. 30 lbs. boneless, skinless chicken breasts

- 10 cans cream of celery soup

- 10 cans cream of mushroom soup

- 5 pkgs. (2 envelopes each) dry onion soup mix

- 3⅓ Tbsp. dried parsley

- 10 small bags of rice or egg noodles

Divine Crock-Pot Chicken

Slow cooker meals are perfect for warm summer days because you don't have to heat up your oven.

5–6 boneless, skinless chicken breasts
1 can cream of celery soup
1 can cream of mushroom soup
1 envelope dry onion soup mix
1 tsp. dried parsley

If freezing, see directions below. Otherwise, place chicken in slow cooker. Mix all other ingredients together and pour over chicken. Cook on low for 4–6 hours. Serve over pasta or rice.

Freezing directions: Place chicken in a gallon-size freezer bag. Pour sauce over chicken. Seal and freeze. You can substitute thin pork chops for the chicken in this recipe. You may want to include a package of rice or egg noodles with this meal.

Easy Chicken Pot Pie

Frozen pie crusts cut your preparation time to almost nothing.

3 boneless, skinless chicken breasts, cooked and diced
1 (16 oz.) bag of frozen mixed vegetables or 2 cups various veggies of
    your choice
1 can cream of chicken soup
¼ cup milk or cream
1 (double) ready-to-bake pie crust
seasonings to taste

Mix together soup and milk until smooth. Stir in veggies. Add chicken and mix. Pour into pie crust. Cover with top crust. Cut 3–6 slits in top of crust. If freezing, see directions below. Otherwise, bake at 400° for 30–40 minutes. Top crust should be golden brown. Cool for 15 minutes before serving.

Freezing directions. Place in a freezer bag or 9×13 disposable aluminum pan; cover with foil and freeze.

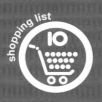

shopping list

- Abt. 15 lbs. boneless, skinless chicken breasts

- 10 bags frozen mixed vegetables

- 10 cans cream of chicken soup

- 2½ cups milk or cream

- 10 double pie crusts

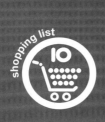

shopping list

- Abt. 30 lbs. boneless, skinless chicken breasts

- 10 cans cream of mushroom soup

- 10 cans cream of chicken soup

- 10 pints sour cream

- 5 lbs. shredded cheddar cheese

- 1 tsp. paprika

- 10 small bags rice or egg noodles

Easy Cheesy Chicken

Simple, creamy, cheesy—a real crowd pleaser.

6 boneless, skinless chicken breasts
1 can cream of mushroom soup
1 can cream of chicken soup
2 cups sour cream
2 cups cheddar cheese
dash of paprika

Place chicken breasts in a greased 9×13 pan. Mix all other ingredients and pour over chicken. If freezing, see directions below. Otherwise, bake uncovered at 350° for 1½–2 hours or until chicken is tender. Serve over rice or egg noodles.

Freezing directions: Place in a disposable aluminum pan and cover with foil. You may want to include a bag of rice or egg noodles with this meal.

Hawaiian Chicken

A sweet way to enjoy your chicken.

6 boneless, skinless chicken breasts
½ cup ketchup
½ tsp. Worcestershire sauce
1 tsp. mustard
½ cup crushed pineapple with juice
½ cup brown sugar

Mix all ingredients together. If freezing, see directions below. Otherwise, bake at 350° for 45 minutes or stew in slow cooker for 4–6 hours. Serve over rice.

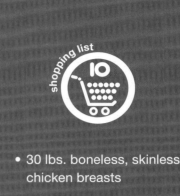

- 30 lbs. boneless, skinless chicken breasts
- 5 cups ketchup
- 5 tsp. Worcestershire sauce
- 10 tsp. mustard
- 2 cans crushed pineapple
- 5 cups brown sugar
- rice

Freezing directions: Place chicken in a freezer bag. Pour sauce mixture over chicken in bag. You may want to include rice with this meal.

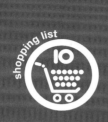

- Abt. 30 lbs. boneless, skinless chicken breasts

- Abt. ⅔ cup dried thyme

- Abt. ⅔ cup salt

- 2 bulbs of garlic

- 10 cups lemon juice (80 oz.)

Lemon Chicken

This chicken has quite the zing! Pair it with Dill-Lemon Rice for a flavorful meal.

6 boneless, skinless chicken breasts
3 tsp. dried thyme
3 tsp. salt
1 clove garlic
1 cup lemon juice

Mix spices and lemon juice in a bag. Add chicken breasts. If freezing, see directions below. Otherwise, marinate for several hours or overnight. Place in slow cooker for 4–6 hours on low. You can also bake or grill instead.

Freezing directions: Place in a freezer bag. The chicken will marinate while thawing.

Dill-Lemon Rice Mix

3 cups long grain rice, uncooked
3 tsp. grated lemon peel
2½ tsp. dill weed
1 tsp. salt
2 Tbsp. instant chicken bouillon powder

Combine all ingredients in a large bowl and blend well. Store in a cool, dry place and use within 6–8 months.

To prepare: Combine Dill–Lemon Rice mix, 4 cups cold water and 2 tablespoons butter or margarine in a medium saucepan. Bring to a boil over high heat. Cover and reduce heat. Simmer for 15–25 minutes until liquid is absorbed.

Freezing directions: Combine ingredients and store in a cool, dry place—no freezing needed.

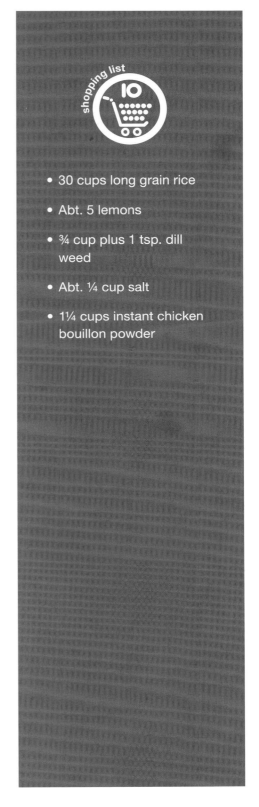

shopping list

- 30 cups long grain rice
- Abt. 5 lemons
- ¾ cup plus 1 tsp. dill weed
- Abt. ¼ cup salt
- 1¼ cups instant chicken bouillon powder

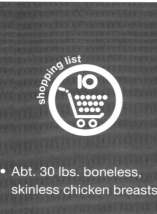

shopping list

- Abt. 30 lbs. boneless, skinless chicken breasts

- 15 cans cream of mushroom soup

- 5 pints sour cream

- 4 boxes Ritz crackers

- 10 cubes butter or margarine

- Abt. 1 cup poppy seeds

Poppy Seed Chicken

The poppy seeds add variety to this chicken casserole.

3 cups cooked and cubed chicken
1½ cans cream of mushroom soup
1 cup sour cream
1½ sleeves Ritz crackers, crushed
1 cube butter or margarine
1½ Tbsp. poppy seeds

Place chicken in the bottom of a greased casserole dish. Mix soup and sour cream. Pour over chicken. Melt butter and stir into crushed crackers. Add poppy seeds and mix together. Spread cracker mixture over chicken. If freezing, see directions below. Otherwise, bake at 375° for 30 minutes.

Freezing directions: Assemble casserole in a disposable aluminum pan. Cover with foil and freeze.

Ritzy Chicken

The crackers give this simple dish a rich flavor.

6 boneless, skinless chicken breasts
2 cups Ritz crackers, crushed (Abt. 45 crackers)
¾ cup shredded mozzarella cheese
¼ tsp. parsley
¼ tsp. salt
⅛ tsp. pepper
⅛ tsp. garlic powder
1 cup melted margarine or butter
⅓ cup apple juice

Mix crackers, cheese and seasonings together. In a separate bowl, mix together margarine and apple juice. Dip chicken in margarine mixture and then coat with cracker mixture. If freezing, see directions below. Otherwise, place in a greased baking dish. Bake at 350° for 1 hour.

Freezing directions: Place in a disposable aluminum pan. Cover with foil and freeze.

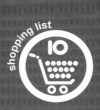

shopping list

- Abt. 30 lbs. boneless, skinless chicken breasts (60 chicken breasts)

- 5 boxes Ritz crackers

- 2 lbs. shredded mozzarella cheese

- 2½ tsp. parsley

- Abt. ½ cup salt

- 1¼ tsp. pepper

- 1¼ tsp. garlic powder

- 20 cubes butter or margarine

- Abt. 1 quart plus 1 pint apple juice (9⅓ cups)

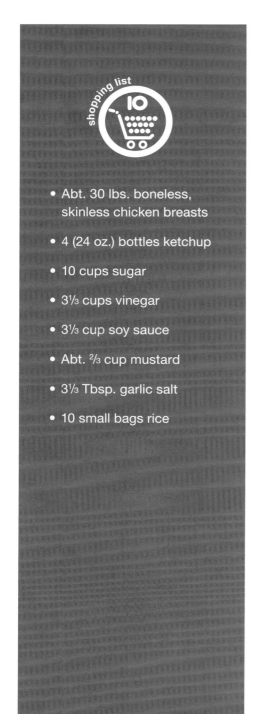
- Abt. 30 lbs. boneless, skinless chicken breasts

- 4 (24 oz.) bottles ketchup

- 10 cups sugar

- 3⅓ cups vinegar

- 3⅓ cup soy sauce

- Abt. ⅔ cup mustard

- 3⅓ Tbsp. garlic salt

- 10 small bags rice

Red Chicken

A tangy, easy way to prepare chicken.

5–6 boneless, skinless chicken breasts
1 cup ketchup
1 cup sugar
⅓ cup vinegar
⅓ cup soy sauce
1 Tbsp. mustard
1 tsp. garlic salt

If freezing, see directions below. Otherwise, place chicken in slow cooker. Mix all other ingredients together and pour over chicken. Cook on low 5–6 hours. Serve over rice.

Freezing directions: Place chicken in a gallon-size freezer bag. Mix all other ingredients together and pour over chicken. Seal and freeze. You may want to include a bag of rice with this meal.

Salsa Chicken

This is also great as a dip for tortilla chips!

4 boneless, skinless chicken breasts
1 (24 oz.) jar salsa
1 (8 oz.) pkg. cream cheese
1 pkg. tortillas

Cook chicken and salsa in slow cooker on high for 3 hours. Shred chicken and add cream cheese. Cook until cream cheese is melted. If freezing, see directions below. Otherwise, spray a frying pan with cooking spray and fry tortillas until browned. Put mixture on tortilla and roll up.

Optional: Add toppings such as lettuce, tomato, olives, and such.

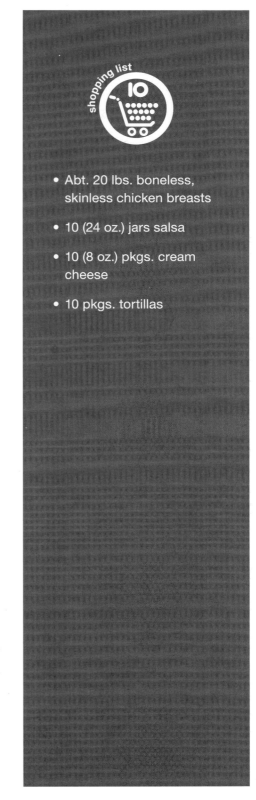

shopping list

10

- Abt. 20 lbs. boneless, skinless chicken breasts

- 10 (24 oz.) jars salsa

- 10 (8 oz.) pkgs. cream cheese

- 10 pkgs. tortillas

Freezing directions: Place in a freezer bag and freeze. Include a bag of tortillas with each meal.

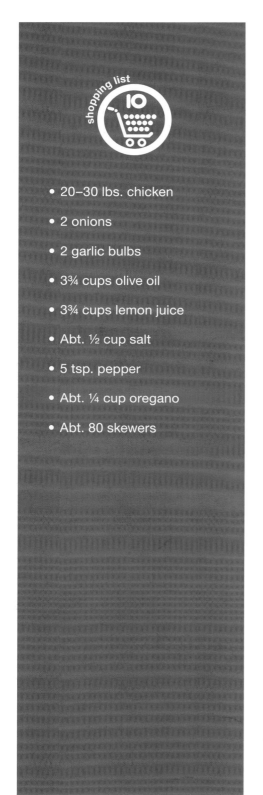

shopping list

10

- 20–30 lbs. chicken

- 2 onions

- 2 garlic bulbs

- 3¾ cups olive oil

- 3¾ cups lemon juice

- Abt. ½ cup salt

- 5 tsp. pepper

- Abt. ¼ cup oregano

- Abt. 80 skewers

Souvlaki Marinated Chicken Skewers

Bring these to your next barbecue and your neighbors will want the recipe.

1 tsp. minced onion
2 cloves garlic, minced
6 Tbsp. olive oil
6 Tbsp. lemon juice
2 tsp. salt
½ tsp. pepper
1 tsp. oregano
2–3 lbs. of chicken, cut in 1- to 2-inch pieces
(can also use pork or turkey)

Combine the onion, garlic, olive oil, lemon juice, salt, pepper, and oregano in a glass bowl or casserole dish. Add the meat and stir well. If freezing, see directions below. Otherwise, cover and marinate in the fridge for 3–4 hours or overnight. Put meat on skewer stick. Cook on a countertop grill or on a barbecue grill. (If you barbecue, soak sticks in water first so they don't catch on fire.) You can also broil until cooked through.

Freezing directions: Place meat in a freezer bag, pour marinade over it, and freeze. The meat will marinate nicely when you thaw it. When thawed, place chicken on skewers.

Stove Top Chicken Casserole

Reminiscent of Thanksgiving dinner . . . but so much easier!

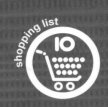

1 box stuffing mix (chicken flavored)
½ cube butter or margarine
2 cups chicken, cooked and diced
1 can cream of chicken soup
1 can cream of celery soup
1 cup milk
2 large stalks of celery washed and sliced

Melt butter. Stir into entire package of stuffing, turning to coat as evenly as possible. Reserve ⅓ of mixture and set aside. Cover the bottom of a 9×13 pan with the stuffing.

Mix all of the other ingredients together and pour over the top of the stuffing. Use the reserved stuffing mix to sprinkle over the top of the casserole. If freezing, see directions below. Otherwise, cover and bake at 350° for 30 minutes or until bubbly. Uncover the last 10 minutes of baking.

Freezing directions: Place in a disposable aluminum pan and cover with foil. You can also use leftover turkey and turkey stuffing for a variation.

shopping list

- 10 boxes stuffing mix (chicken flavored)

- 5 cubes butter or margarine

- Abt. 20 lbs chicken breasts

- 10 cans cream of chicken soup

- 10 cans cream of celery soup

- 10 cups milk

- 20 stalks of celery

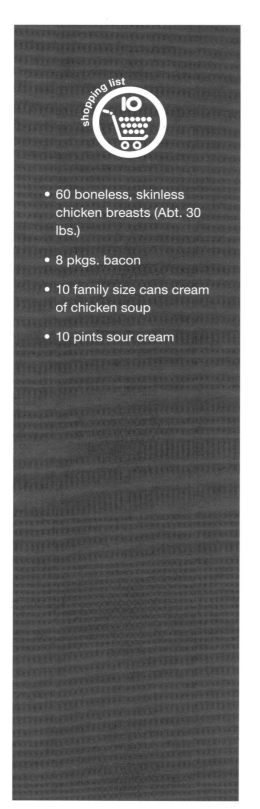

- 60 boneless, skinless chicken breasts (Abt. 30 lbs.)

- 8 pkgs. bacon

- 10 family size cans cream of chicken soup

- 10 pints sour cream

Sunday Chicken

A perfect Sunday meal—it bakes long enough for everyone to enjoy church, then come home to the wonderful smell of Sunday dinner!

6 boneless, skinless chicken breasts
12 slices bacon
1 family size can cream of chicken soup
1 pint sour cream

Place chicken in pan. Cover with bacon slices. Mix soup and sour cream together. Pour over chicken and bacon. If freezing, see directions below. Otherwise, cover and bake at 325° for 3 hours. Serve over rice.

Freezing directions: Cover tightly with foil. Freeze in a disposable aluminum pan. You may want to include rice with this meal.

Sweet and Sour Chicken

This meal has just the right tang!

4–5 boneless, skinless chicken breasts
1 small onion, chopped
½ cup soy sauce
½ cup vinegar
⅔ cup white sugar
1 green bell pepper, chopped in 1-inch pieces
2–3 carrots, sliced
½ cup ketchup
1 Tbsp. cornstarch
1 (15 oz.) can pineapple chunks

Cut up chicken into 1-inch pieces and brown in onions and soy sauce. Add vinegar, sugar, and the juice from the pineapple chunks (save chunks for later). Add vegetables. Stir in ketchup. Mix cornstarch with ¼ cup water. Add to mixture and stir until thick; add pineapple. If freezing, see directions below. Otherwise, serve over rice.

 Freezing directions: Pour into a freezer bag and freeze. You may want to include a bag of rice with this meal.

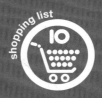

shopping list

- Abt. 25 lbs. boneless, skinless chicken breasts
- 10 small onions
- 5 cups soy sauce
- 5 cups vinegar
- 6⅔ cups white sugar
- 10 green bell peppers
- 20–30 carrots
- 5 cups ketchup
- 10 Tbsp. cornstarch
- 10 cans pineapple chunks
- 10 bags rice

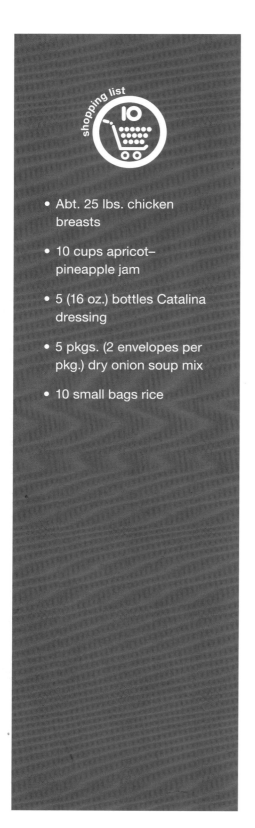

- Abt. 25 lbs. chicken breasts

- 10 cups apricot–pineapple jam

- 5 (16 oz.) bottles Catalina dressing

- 5 pkgs. (2 envelopes per pkg.) dry onion soup mix

- 10 small bags rice

Sweet Chicken

This will be a family favorite.

6–8 boneless skinless chicken breasts
1 cup apricot-pineapple jam
1 cup Catalina dressing
¼ cup dry onion soup mix

Put chicken breasts in a 9×13 pan. Mix all other ingredients together and pour over chicken. If freezing, see directions below. Otherwise, cover and cook 1½ to 2 hours or until chicken is done. Serve over rice.

Freezing directions: You can freeze this in a freezer bag, or a disposable aluminum pan. You can also prepare in a slow cooker for 4–5 hours. You may want to include a package of rice with this meal.

Swiss Chicken

Pull this out of your freezer to impress drop-in-company.

6–8 boneless, skinless chicken breasts
12–16 slices Swiss cheese
2 cans cream of mushroom soup
⅓ cup water
½ cup seasoned bread crumbs
¼ cup melted butter

Place chicken breasts in a greased 9×13 pan. Top each breast with 2 slices of Swiss cheese. Mix soup and water and pour over chicken and cheese. Sprinkle bread crumbs over top; then drizzle melted butter over bread crumbs. If freezing, see directions below. Otherwise, bake at 350° for 1½ hours or until chicken is tender.

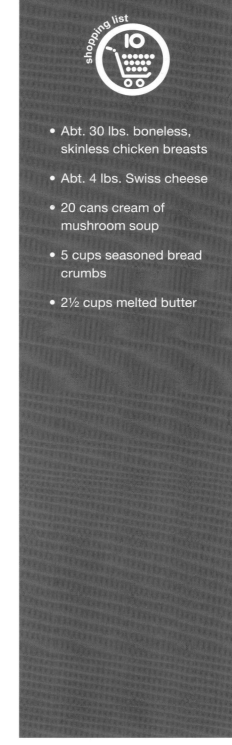

shopping list

- Abt. 30 lbs. boneless, skinless chicken breasts
- Abt. 4 lbs. Swiss cheese
- 20 cans cream of mushroom soup
- 5 cups seasoned bread crumbs
- 2½ cups melted butter

Freezing directions: If you are using frozen chicken, omit the water in the recipe. To freeze, place in a disposable aluminum pan. Cover and freeze.

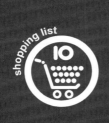

Shopping List

- 60 boneless, skinless chicken breast (Abt. 30 lbs.)
- 10 medium onions
- 20 cloves garlic
- 1¼ cups balsamic vinegar
- 1¼ cup instant chicken bouillon powder
- 2½ tsp. crushed red pepper
- 1 tsp. dried oregano
- 30 cups long grain rice
- 20 tomatoes

Oregano Chicken

It is possible to include meals with fresh produce. Keep the produce in the fridge and use this Make-Ahead Meal early in the month.

6 boneless, skinless chicken breasts
1 medium onion, cut into wedges
2 cloves garlic
2 Tbsp. balsamic vinegar
2 tsp. instant chicken bouillon powder
2 cups water
1 tsp. dried oregano
¼ tsp. crushed red pepper
2 tomatoes, sliced
6 cups cooked rice

If freezing, see directions below. Otherwise, in slow cooker, combine onion and garlic. Add the chicken breasts. In a bowl, stir together water, balsamic vinegar, bouillon, oregano, and crushed red pepper. Pour over chicken and cook on low for 5–6 hours or high for 3 hours. Place 1 cup of rice on plate and place some tomato slices on top of rice. Place cooked chicken on top of rice and tomato and serve.

Freezing directions: Mix all ingredients together and place in a gallon-size freezer bag. Include in separate sandwich bags 3 cups of long grain rice and 2 fresh tomatoes (don't freeze the tomatoes).

Teriyaki Chicken Stir-fry

Healthy and simple—what a great combination!

1½ lbs of boneless skinless chicken breasts, sliced into strips (you can also use chicken tenderloin strips), marinated in teriyaki sauce (see recipe below)
1 bag of frozen stir-fry vegetables
cooked rice
chow mein noodles

Teriyaki marinade:

½ tsp. ginger
2 tsp. dry mustard
¼ cup of oil (any kind)
½ cup soy sauce (lite or reduced salt also works fine)
1 tsp. garlic
2 Tbsp. molasses

Combine all marinade ingredients. Put chicken strips in a container and pour marinade over. If freezing, see directions below. Otherwise, let it sit in the fridge overnight or for several hours to marinate. To prepare, pour chicken and marinade into a large skillet. Cook until meat is cooked through and marinade boils for at least 5 minutes (to kill any bacteria from chicken). Add in the vegetables and stir constantly until done. Serve over cooked rice and top with chow mein noodles.

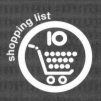

shopping list

- 15 lbs boneless skinless chicken breasts or chicken tenderloins

- 10 pkgs. of frozen stir-fry vegetables

- 2½ tsp. ginger

- ⅓ c. + 2 tsp. of dry mustard

- 2½ cups oil

- 5 cups soy sauce

- 3 Tbsp. + 2 tsp. garlic

- 1¼ c. molasses

- 30 cups long grain rice

- 20 cups chow mein noodles

Freezing directions: Place meat and marinade in a freezer bag. To prepare, thaw meat in the refrigerator and prepare as recipe states, or place in a slow cooker for 2–3 hours. When chicken is done, add to skillet with vegetables and stir-fry.

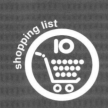

- Abt. 30 lbs. of chicken breasts (60 chicken breasts)

- Abt. ¼ cup seasoned salt

- Abt. ¼ cup garlic salt

- 2½ cups brown sugar

- Abt. 1½ cup of flour

- 5 onions

- 5 red bell peppers

- 5 green bell peppers

- 10 large cans stewed tomatoes

- 10 cans tomato soup

- Abt. ½ cup Worcestershire sauce

- 10 small bags rice

Tomato Chicken

A flavorful meal.

6 chicken breasts
1 tsp. seasoned salt
1 tsp. garlic salt
¼ cup brown sugar
2 Tbsp. flour
½ sliced onion
½ red bell pepper
½ green pepper
2 (15 oz.) cans stewed tomatoes (or 1 large can)
1 can tomato soup
⅔ soup can of water
2 tsp. Worcestershire sauce

Line a 9×13 pan with chicken breasts. Sprinkle chicken with seasonings, sugar, and flour. Top with onion and peppers. In a separate bowl, mix together stewed tomatoes, tomato soup, water, and Worcestershire sauce. Pour mixture over chicken. If freezing, see directions below. Otherwise, cover with foil and bake covered at 325° for 2–2½ hours. (This also works well in a slow cooker.) Serve over cooked rice.

Freezing directions: Place ingredients in order in a disposable aluminum pan, cover with plastic wrap and then with foil and freeze. Or, to prepare in slow cooker, place all ingredients in a freezer bag. You may want to include a bag of rice with this meal.

Pork Recipes

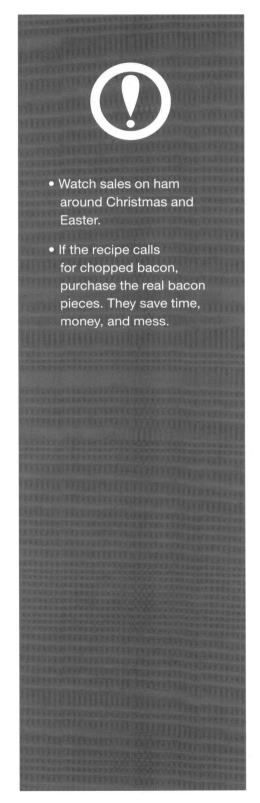

- Watch sales on ham around Christmas and Easter.

- If the recipe calls for chopped bacon, purchase the real bacon pieces. They save time, money, and mess.

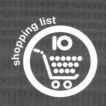

shopping list

- 10 pkgs. shredded frozen hash browns

- 10 pkgs. cooked crumbled bacon, or Abt. 10 pkgs. raw bacon

- 10 pints sour cream

- 5 cups butter or margarine

- 5 lbs. shredded cheddar cheese

- 5 bunches green onions

- 5 cups seasoned bread crumbs

Baked Potato Casserole

Baked potato taste in a casserole!

1 pkg. frozen shredded hash browns
1 cup cooked and crumbled bacon (or precooked bacon bits, not imitation)
1 pint sour cream
½ cup butter or margarine, divided
2 cups shredded cheddar cheese
½ cup chopped green onions
½ cup seasoned bread crumbs

Mix together hash browns, bacon, sour cream, ¼ cup melted butter, cheese, and onions. Place in a 9×13 pan. Sprinkle with bread crumbs and top with remaining dabs of butter. If freezing, see directions below. Otherwise, bake at 375° for 1 hour.

Freezing directions: Place in a disposable aluminum pan and cover with foil.

Breakfast Burritos

These make a quick and easy breakfast, lunch, or dinner!
Great for lunches on the go!

1 to 1½ lbs. of ground sausage, cooked and drained
12–18 eggs, scrambled (salt and pepper to taste)
1 cup shredded cheddar cheese
1 cup shredded pepper jack cheese
8 burrito size flour tortillas

Warm tortillas in microwave to soften. Fill each tortilla with ¼ cup cheese (half cheddar, half pepper jack), ½ cup eggs, and ¼ cup sausage. Wrap into a burrito and then wrap in foil. If freezing, see directions below. Otherwise, bake in the foil at 350° for 10–15 minutes until cheese is melted and they are heated through. (Rotate halfway through baking time.) You may also choose to warm on a barbecue grill. Make sure they are fully thawed for this method. Place wrapped burrito on grill. Rotate and turn often until they are warm throughout and the cheese is melted. You may also heat in a microwave for quick lunches, but the tortilla will not be browned and crispy.

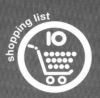

- 10–15 lbs. ground sausage, cooked and drained

- 10–15 dozen eggs

- 2½ lbs. shredded cheddar cheese

- 2½ lbs. shredded pepper jack cheese

- 80 burrito size tortillas

Freezing directions: Place wrapped burritos in a freezer bag and freeze.

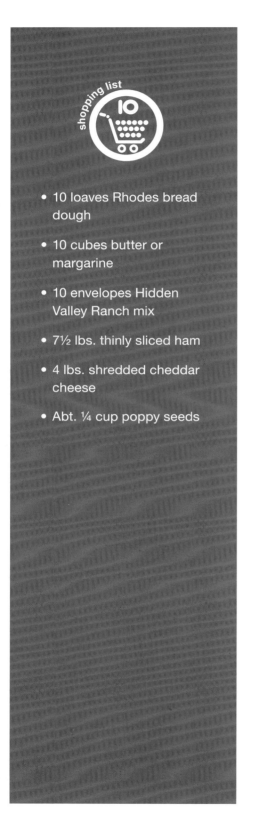

shopping list

- 10 loaves Rhodes bread dough

- 10 cubes butter or margarine

- 10 envelopes Hidden Valley Ranch mix

- 7½ lbs. thinly sliced ham

- 4 lbs. shredded cheddar cheese

- Abt. ¼ cup poppy seeds

Brunch Braid

If you blink, you might not get any of this fabulous bread!

1 loaf Rhodes bread dough
1 cube butter or margarine
1 envelope Hidden Valley Ranch mix (not generic)
¾ lb. thinly sliced ham
1½ cups shredded cheddar cheese
1 tsp. poppy seeds

Roll bread dough out into a rectangular shape so it's approximately ½ inch thick. Combine margarine and ranch mix. Spread about 5 tablespoons of mixture on the rectangle. Layer ham and cheese down the center of rectangle. Use a pizza cutter to cut strips along each side of the dough (even numbers on each side). Starting at the bottom, take each piece, cross, and twist. Continue crisscrossing until your pizza is braided. Carefully place on a greased cookie sheet. Brush remaining butter/ranch mixture over top. Sprinkle with poppy seeds. If freezing, see directions below. Otherwise, bake at 350° for 25 to 30 minutes.

Freezing directions: Wrap loaf with plastic wrap and then foil.

Cheesy Funeral Potatoes with Ham

A classic, and it's perfect for around Easter!

1 (2 lb.) bag frozen, cubed, or shredded hash browns
1 family size can of cream of mushroom or cream of chicken soup
1 cup fat free plain yogurt or sour cream
2 Tbsp. parsley
2 Tbsp. dried onions
2 cups shredded cheddar cheese
sliced ham

Mix all ingredients together. If freezing, see directions below. Otherwise, place in a 9×13 pan and bake at 350° for 1 hour. Serve this with sliced ham.

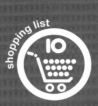

shopping list

- 10 (2 lbs.) bags frozen, cubed, or shredded hash browns

- 10 family size cans cream of mushroom or cream of chicken soup

- 5 pints plain yogurt or sour cream (can use fat free)

- 1¼ cups parsley

- 1¼ cups dried onion

- 5 lbs. shredded cheddar cheese

- Abt. 4 whole boneless hams, dinner sliced

Freezing directions: Place in a disposable aluminum pan. Place 10–12 slices of ham in a freezer bag and include with the pan of potatoes to make this a meal.

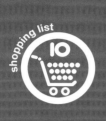

shopping list

- 10 tubes refrigerator crescent rolls

- 10 lbs. ground sausage

- 5 lbs. shredded Monterey Jack cheese

- 5 dozen eggs

- 5 green bell peppers (optional)

- 10 cups milk

Crescent Roll Breakfast Casserole

Breakfast for dinner! Ya gotta love it!

1 (8 oz.) tube refrigerator crescent rolls
1 lb. ground sausage, cooked and well drained
2 cups shredded Monterey Jack cheese
6 eggs, beaten
3 Tbsp. minced green bell pepper (optional)
1 cup milk
salt and pepper to taste

Beat together eggs, milk, salt, and pepper. Stir in cheese and green pepper and mix well. Set aside. Unroll tube of crescent rolls and press together to cover the bottom of a 9×13 pan. Seal perforations. Crumble cooked sausage over rolls. Pour egg mixture over rolls and sausage. If freezing, see directions below. Otherwise, refrigerate overnight if cooking it in the morning or bake at 425° for 20 to 25 minutes until browned.

Freezing directions: Prepare in a disposable aluminum pan that has been sprayed with cooking spray. Cover with foil.

Green Bean and Bacon Casserole

We were surprised that even our kids loved this vegetable-based dish

12 oz. bacon (or use pre-cooked bacon bits, not artificial)
1 small onion, chopped
1½ cups diced carrots
3 cups peeled and diced potatoes
1 can green beans
2 Tbsp. butter or margarine (can replace with bacon drippings for added
    flavor)
¼ cup flour
3 cups milk
1 tsp. salt
¼ tsp. pepper
2 cups shredded cheese, divided

Brown bacon and onion. Cut bacon into 1-inch pieces. Boil potatoes and carrots until tender. Set aside. In a medium saucepan, melt butter. Add flour and mix together. Slowly pour in milk and stir constantly with a whisk until thick and bubbly. Add salt, pepper, and 1½ cups of cheese. Mix all ingredients together. If freezing, see directions below. Otherwise, place in a 9×13 baking dish. Sprinkle with remaining cheese and bake at 350° for 30 minutes.

 Freezing directions: Slightly undercook potatoes. Place in a disposable aluminum pan, or cool and put into a freezer bag. Include shredded cheese for topping.

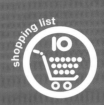

shopping list

- 10 pkgs. bacon
- 10 small onions
- 40 carrots
- 40 potatoes
- 10 cans green beans
- 20 cups shredded cheese (5 lbs.)
- 2 gallons milk
- Abt. ¼ cup salt
- 2½ tsp. pepper
- 2½ cups flour
- 1¼ cup butter or margarine

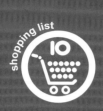
- 5 cubes margarine
- Abt. 20 stalks celery
- 5 onions
- 20 cups ketchup
- 1¼ cups vinegar
- 1¼ cups lemon juice
- 2½ cups Worcestershire Sauce
- 2½ cups brown sugar
- Abt. ½ cup dry mustard
- Abt. ¼ cup pepper
- 10 cans tomato soup
- Abt. 3 whole hams, sliced wafer thin
- 10 pkgs. buns or hard rolls

Ham Barbecue

A terrific recipe—great for large family gatherings.

¼ cup margarine or butter
1 cup chopped celery
½ onion, chopped
1 cup water
2 cups ketchup
2 Tbsp. vinegar
2 Tbsp. lemon juice
¼ cup Worcestershire sauce
¼ cup brown sugar
2 tsp. dry mustard
1 tsp. pepper
1 can tomato soup

Wafer sliced ham (enough to make 8 sandwiches; the sauce goes a long way so you could add more if you like)

Sauté chopped celery and chopped onion together in margarine. Add the rest of the ingredients and cook together for about 15 minutes or until heated through.

If freezing, see directions below. Otherwise, pour sauce over ham in a baking dish and bake at 300° for 30–40 minutes or in a slow cooker on low 3–4 hours. Serve on buns or hard rolls.

Freezing directions: Cool. Place ham in a freezer bag and pour sauce over. Include a bag of buns or hard rolls with this meal.

Ham Biscuits

Another kid favorite!

2 cups ham, chopped
1 Tbsp. mustard
1 Tbsp. melted butter
dash of garlic salt
2 cans refrigerator biscuits
8 slices cheddar cheese

Mix ham, mustard, butter, and garlic salt together. Flatten a biscuit to ¼ inch thick. Put ¼ cup of ham mixture on the biscuit and put a slice of cheese on top of the ham mixture. Top with another flattened biscuit and seal the sides. If freezing, see directions below. Otherwise, place on a cookie sheet and bake at 350° for 12–15 minutes until golden brown.

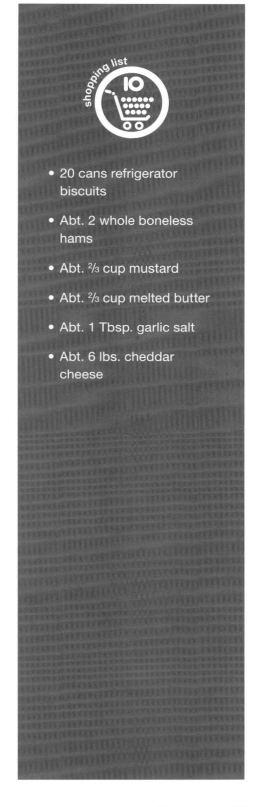

shopping list 10

- 20 cans refrigerator biscuits

- Abt. 2 whole boneless hams

- Abt. ⅔ cup mustard

- Abt. ⅔ cup melted butter

- Abt. 1 Tbsp. garlic salt

- Abt. 6 lbs. cheddar cheese

Freezing directions: Flash freeze. Remove from freezer and place in freezer bags (4–6 to a gallon-size bag).

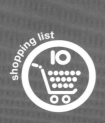

shopping list

10

- 10 dozen eggs

- 10 (12 oz.) cans evaporated milk

- Abt. ¼ cup salt

- 5 tsp. pepper

- 10 pkgs. shredded hash browns

- 25 cups shredded cheese (6½ lbs.)

- 10 small onions

- 10 medium green peppers

- 20 cups ham, cubed (Abt. 2 whole fully cooked hams)

Hash Brown Casserole

This makes a great weekend breakfast. Or our favorite: breakfast for dinner!

12 eggs
1 (12 oz.) can evaporated milk
½ tsp. salt
½ tsp. pepper
1 pkg. shredded hash browns
2½ cups shredded cheddar cheese (divided)
1 small onion, chopped
1 medium green pepper, chopped
2 cups ham, cubed

In a large bowl, combine eggs, milk, salt, and pepper. Stir in the hash browns, 1½ cups cheese, onion, green pepper, and ham. Pour in a greased 9×13 baking dish. If freezing, see directions below. Otherwise, bake uncovered at 350° for 60–75 minutes, or until a knife inserted near the center comes out clean. Should be moist because of cheese, but not runny. Top with remaining cheese and let melt.

Freezing directions: Place in a greased disposable aluminum pan. Place 1 cup of the shredded cheese in a bag and freeze along with casserole to be sprinkled on after baking.

Ham and Cornbread Casserole

It's hard to believe that something so simple can be so delicious!

2 eggs
1 (16 oz.) can cream style corn
1 (16 oz.) can whole kernel corn
½ cup butter or margarine, melted
1 cup sour cream
1 pkg. corn muffin mix (Jiffy)
2 cups cubed ham
1 cup shredded cheddar cheese

Beat eggs. Stir in cream corn, whole kernel corn, butter, and sour cream. Add muffin mix and ham. Pour into a greased 9×13 pan. If freezing, see directions below. Otherwise, Bake at 375° for 45 minutes or until center is done. Take out and sprinkle cheese on top. Return to oven until cheese is melted.

shopping list

- 20 eggs
- 10 (16 oz.) cans cream style corn
- 10 (16 oz.) cans whole kernel corn
- 10 cubes butter or margarine
- 5 pints sour cream
- 10 pkgs. corn muffin mix (Jiffy)
- 2 whole boneless hams
- 3 lbs. shredded cheddar cheese

Freezing directions: Freeze it in a disposable aluminum pan and cover with foil. Include 1 cup shredded cheese in a bag to sprinkle on after baking.

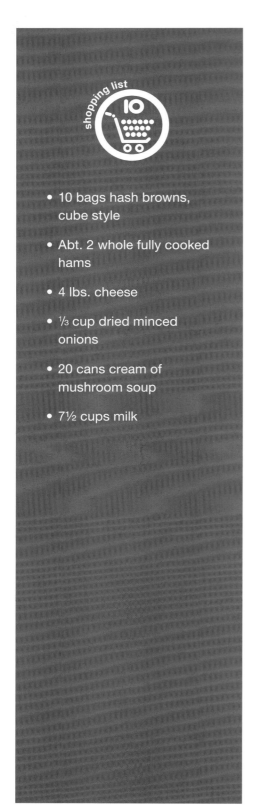

- 10 bags hash browns, cube style
- Abt. 2 whole fully cooked hams
- 4 lbs. cheese
- 1/3 cup dried minced onions
- 20 cans cream of mushroom soup
- 7½ cups milk

Ham and Potato Casserole

This is a wonderful brunch recipe. Pair it with a fruit salad to "wow" a crowd!

1 bag frozen hash browns, cube style
2 cups cubed ham
1½ cups cubed cheddar cheese (can also mix this with mozzarella)
1 Tbsp. dried minced onions
2 cans cream of mushroom soup
¾ cup milk
salt and pepper to taste
1½ cups shredded cheese

Mix all ingredients except cheese together and place in a 9×13 casserole dish. If freezing, see directions below. Otherwise, cover with foil and bake at 375° for 1–1½ hours or until potatoes are done. Remove foil and sprinkle with shredded cheese and put back in oven until melted.

Freezing directions: Place in a disposable aluminum pan and cover with foil. Include cheese to sprinkle on top.

Ham and Swiss Casserole

Whip this up anytime for a satisfying meal.

1 (8 oz.) pkg. wide egg noodles, cooked and drained
2 cups ham, cubed
2 cups Swiss cheese, shredded
1 can cream of mushroom soup
1 cup sour cream

In a 9×13 pan, layer noodles, ham, and cheese; mix lightly. In a separate bowl, mix the soup and sour cream together. Pour soup mixture over the other ingredients in the pan. If freezing, see directions below. Otherwise, bake at 350° for 45 minutes. Cover during the first half of baking.

shopping list

- 10 (8 oz.) pkgs. of wide egg noodles
- Abt. 2 whole cooked hams
- 20 cups shredded Swiss cheese
- 10 cans cream of mushroom soup
- 5 pints sour cream

Freezing directions: Slightly undercook the noodles. Place in a disposable aluminum pan and cover with foil.

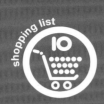
- 40 stalks celery
- 10 green peppers
- 10 onions
- 10 (16 oz.) pkgs. frozen peas
- 10 cans cream of mushroom soup
- 10 cans cream of chicken soup
- 1¼ cups soy sauce
- 10 cups rice
- 10 cans bean sprouts
- 7½ cups slivered almonds
- Abt. 20 cups chow mein noodles

Oriental Casserole

Don't order out for Chinese! Pull this out of your freezer for a sure-fire hit.

1 lb. link sausages (browned ground beef may be substituted)
2 cups sliced celery
1 green pepper, chopped (optional)
1 onion, chopped
1 (16 oz.) pkg. frozen peas (optional)
1 can cream of mushroom soup
1 can cream of chicken soup
1 cup water
2 Tbsp. soy sauce
3 cups cooked rice
1 can bean sprouts, drained and rinsed
¾ cup slivered almonds
chow mein noodles

Slice the link sausages ¼ inch thick. In a frying pan, cook sausage until browned. Drain off most of the fat. Set aside. Sauté celery, green pepper, and onion until tender. Mix with sausage. Add peas, soups, water, soy sauce, rice, and bean sprouts. Put in a 9×13 casserole dish and sprinkle with slivered almonds. If freezing, see directions below. Otherwise, cover and bake at 350° for 30–40 minutes.

Serve over cooked rice and top with chow mein noodles, or just serve over chow mein noodles.

Freezing directions: Place in a disposable aluminum pan, and cover tightly with foil. Place chow mein noodles aside, or freeze separately to use on top when serving. For your group, you may include a small package of rice and a bag of chow mein noodles to serve with.

Pizza and Pasta

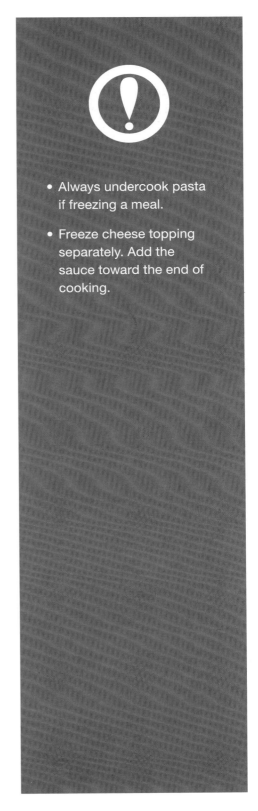

- Always undercook pasta if freezing a meal.

- Freeze cheese topping separately. Add the sauce toward the end of cooking.

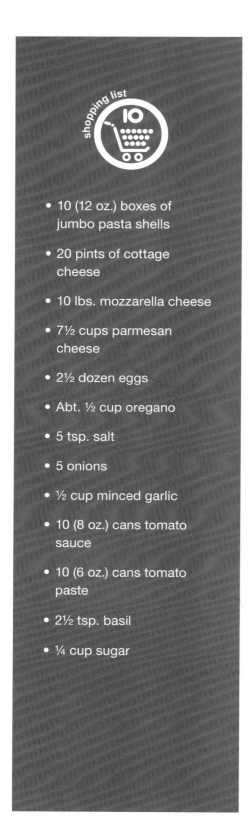

- 10 (12 oz.) boxes of jumbo pasta shells
- 20 pints of cottage cheese
- 10 lbs. mozzarella cheese
- 7½ cups parmesan cheese
- 2½ dozen eggs
- Abt. ½ cup oregano
- 5 tsp. salt
- 5 onions
- ½ cup minced garlic
- 10 (8 oz.) cans tomato sauce
- 10 (6 oz.) cans tomato paste
- 2½ tsp. basil
- ¼ cup sugar

Cheese-Filled Shells

Kids love to fill these shells almost as much as they love to eat them!

1 (12 oz.) box jumbo pasta shells

Cheese Mixture:
2 pints cottage cheese
1 lb. shredded mozzarella cheese
¾ cup parmesan cheese
3 eggs
¾ tsp. oregano
½ tsp. salt

Sauce:
½ cup diced onion
2 tsp. minced garlic
1 (8 oz.) can tomato sauce
1 (6 oz.) can tomato paste
1 cup water
1 tsp. oregano
¼ tsp. basil
1 tsp. sugar

Cook shells half of recommended time, just until limp. Drain and cool in a single layer on a pan. Combine cheese, eggs, oregano, and salt. Fill a quart-size freezer bag with cheese mixture and snip off corner. Squeeze out mixture into shells. Cover and put in refrigerator while preparing sauce. Combine all of the sauce ingredients and simmer 1 hour in a saucepan. If freezing, see directions below. Otherwise, pour ½ cup of sauce in the bottom of a baking dish. Place shells in a single layer in the baking dish. Cover with the rest of the sauce. Bake at 350° for 30 minutes.

Freezing directions: After filling the shells, flash freeze them. Place them in a freezer bag. Pour sauce in a separate freezer bag and freeze.

Cheesy Rigatoni Bake

A mild Italian dish that goes well with a salad and garlic bread.

1 (16 oz.) pkg. rigatoni noodles
2 Tbsp. butter or margarine
¼ cup flour
½ tsp. salt
2 cups milk
¼ cup water
4 eggs, beaten
2 (8 oz.) cans tomato sauce
2 cups shredded mozzarella cheese
¼ cup shredded parmesan cheese

Cook pasta according to package directions. In a saucepan, melt butter. Stir in flour and salt until smooth, gradually add milk and water. Bring to a boil, cook and stir for 2 minutes or until thickened.

Drain pasta and place in a large bowl. Add beaten eggs. Spoon into a greased 9×13 pan. Top with tomato sauce and mozzarella cheese. Spoon white sauce over top and sprinkle with parmesan cheese. If freezing, see directions below. Otherwise, bake at 375° for 30 to 35 minutes.

Freezing directions: Slightly undercook pasta. Place in a greased disposable aluminum pan. Cover with plastic wrap and then aluminum foil.

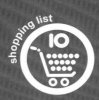

shopping list

- 10 (16 oz.) pkgs. rigatoni noodles
- 1¼ cup butter or margarine
- 2½ cups flour
- Abt. 2 Tbsp. salt
- 1 gallon plus 1 quart milk
- 3 dozen plus 4 eggs
- 20 (8 oz.) cans tomato sauce
- 5 lbs. shredded mozzarella cheese
- 2½ cups shredded parmesan cheese

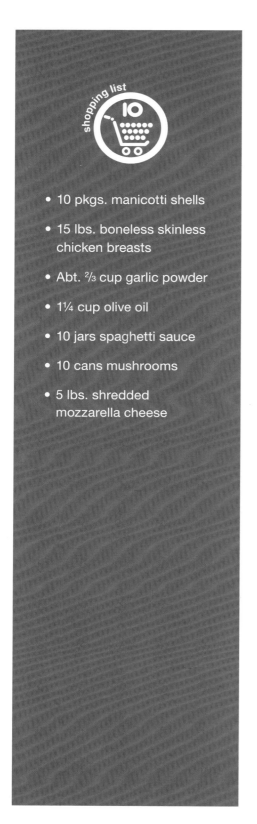

shopping list
10

- 10 pkgs. manicotti shells

- 15 lbs. boneless skinless chicken breasts

- Abt. ⅔ cup garlic powder

- 1¼ cup olive oil

- 10 jars spaghetti sauce

- 10 cans mushrooms

- 5 lbs. shredded mozzarella cheese

Chicken Manicotti

Using uncooked manicotti shells makes this recipe a snap to put together.

2 Tbsp. olive oil
1 Tbsp. garlic powder
1½ lbs. boneless, skinless chicken breasts
10 uncooked manicotti shells
1 jar spaghetti sauce, divided
1 can mushrooms
2 cups shredded mozzarella cheese
⅔ cup water

Cut chicken into 1-inch strips and brown in olive oil and garlic powder. Spread 1 cup of spaghetti sauce in a 9×13 pan. Stuff chicken into uncooked manicotti shells and place on top of spaghetti sauce. Top shells with mushrooms and pour remaining sauce over the top. Sprinkle with cheese. Pour water around the edges of the dish. If freezing, see directions below. Otherwise, cover and bake at 375° for 50–60 minutes or until pasta is tender.

Freezing directions: Place in a disposable aluminum pan, cover with plastic wrap and then foil. Remove plastic wrap and re-cover with foil before baking.

Homemade Pizza

Who couldn't use a pizza in the freezer?

2 cups flour
2 tsp. active dry yeast
1 tsp. sugar
½ tsp. salt
¾ cup warm water
2 Tbsp. olive oil
pizza sauce
toppings

Dissolve yeast and sugar in warm water in a measuring cup; let stand until bubbly—about 10 minutes. Stir in olive oil and salt. Place flour in a mixing bowl and add yeast mixture. Mix all together until the dough forms a ball. Place dough in a greased bowl and cover with plastic wrap that has been sprayed with cooking spray. Let rise until double—about 1–1½ hours. When ready, roll out on pizza pan. If freezing, see directions below. Otherwise, top with sauce and toppings that your family likes. Bake at 375° for 20–25 minutes. Watch crust and check often.

Freezing directions: After rolling out, flash freeze crust. Remove from pan and wrap in plastic. Then cover with foil and freeze. You can freeze shredded mozzarella cheese and the meats to put on the pizza along with it. If you make homemade pizza sauce, you may freeze that as well or put the toppings on the pizza and freeze it that way.

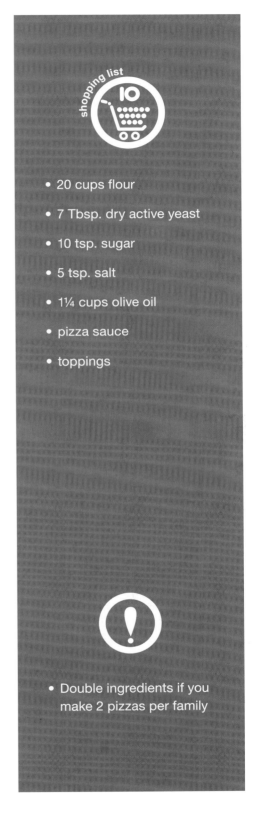

shopping list

- 20 cups flour
- 7 Tbsp. dry active yeast
- 10 tsp. sugar
- 5 tsp. salt
- 1¼ cups olive oil
- pizza sauce
- toppings

- Double ingredients if you make 2 pizzas per family

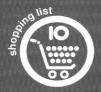

shopping list

10

- 15 lbs. ground beef
- ¾ cup parsley
- 7 Tbsp. + 1½ tsp. salt
- 30 (6 oz.) cans tomato paste
- 5 tsp. garlic powder
- Abt. ¼ cup basil
- 10 (15 oz.) cans Italian stewed tomatoes
- 10 (8 oz.) cans tomato sauce
- 10 large containers cottage cheese
- 20 eggs
- 5 tsp. pepper
- 10 lbs. shredded mozzarella cheese
- 7 (16 oz.) pkgs. lasagna noodles

Lasagna

No need to use no-bake noodles or even boil the noodles if you are freezing it! The moisture in the lasagna and the freezing and thawing process takes care of it!

Sauce:
1½ lbs. ground beef, browned and drained
1½ tsp. parsley
1¼ tsp. salt
3 (6 oz.) cans tomato paste
½ tsp. garlic powder
1 tsp. basil
1 (15 oz.) can Italian stewed tomatoes
1 (8 oz.) can tomato sauce

Cheese filling:
3 cups cottage cheese
2 tsp. parsley
1 tsp. salt
2 eggs, beaten
1 cup shredded parmesan cheese
½ tsp. pepper
4 cups shredded mozzarella cheese
12 lasagna noodles, cooked according to pkg. (or use non-cook kind)

Combine sauce ingredients together in a large saucepan. Simmer 15 minutes. Mix together all cheese filling ingredients. Place noodles to cover the bottom of a 9×13 pan. Spread ½ the cheese filling over the noodles and sprinkle 2 cups of cheese on top. Spread sauce over that and repeat layers one more time. If freezing, see directions below. Otherwise, bake at 375° for 30–45 minutes until bubbly. Let sit for 15 minutes before serving.

Freezing directions: If preparing in bulk, do in assembly style. Place dry noodles (no need to boil the noodles if freezing) in all the pans, top with cheese in all the pans, etc. It helps also if you prepare the meat filling one day and let it cool in the fridge before you assemble. Freeze in a disposable aluminum pan and cover with plastic wrap and then foil.

Lasagna Rolls

If you have a lasagna-loving family, this will top your list!

9 lasagna noodles, cooked and cooled
1 jar spaghetti sauce, divided

Filling:
1 (24 oz.) container of cottage cheese
1 egg
¼ cup parmesan cheese
1 Tbsp. parsley flakes
⅛ tsp. black pepper
1 tsp. garlic salt
½ cup frozen spinach (optional)
3 cups shredded mozzarella cheese, divided

Pour half of the spaghetti sauce in a 9×13 baking dish. Mix together all ingredients of the filling except 1 cup of the mozzarella cheese. Place 1 lasagna noodle on a cutting board and spread the entire length of the noodle with filling. Roll up like a sleeping bag and lay in pan. Continue until all 9 noodles are rolled. Top with remaining sauce and mozzarella cheese. If freezing, see directions below. Otherwise, bake at 350° for 30–40 minutes.

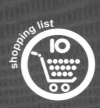

shopping list

10

- 5 lbs. lasagna noodles

- 10 jars spaghetti sauce

- 10 large containers cottage cheese

- 10 eggs

- 2½ cups parmesan cheese

- ⅔ cup parsley flakes

- 1 Tbsp. black pepper

- ¼ cup garlic salt

- 5 cups spinach

- 30 cups mozzarella cheese (Abt. 8 lbs.)

Freezing directions: Slightly undercook the noodles. Place in a disposable aluminum pan and cover with plastic wrap and then foil. If you cook from frozen, keep pan covered for the first half of baking.

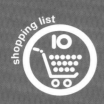

- 10 pkgs. of yeast (⅔ cup)

- ⅔ cup sugar

- 9 Tbsp. salt

- 2½ cups oil

- Abt. 20 cups flour

- 5 jars spaghetti sauce

- 20 lbs. shredded mozzarella cheese

- 2 cubes butter

- 5 tsp. garlic salt

- 1¼ cups parmesan cheese

Pizza Braids

A family favorite—these take some extra time, but the family will love you for it!

Dough:
>1 cup warm water
>1 pkg. yeast
>1 Tbsp. sugar
>¾ tsp. salt
>¼ cup oil
>2 cups flour

Topping:
>½ jar spaghetti sauce
>3–4 cups shredded mozzarella cheese
>pizza toppings (whatever kind your family likes)
>1½ Tbsp. butter
>½ tsp. garlic salt
>2 Tbsp. parmesan cheese

Mix together all dough ingredients. Dough should be slightly sticky to the touch—not too stiff, just a nice, workable dough. Roll out on a floured surface into a rectangular shape. Add the toppings.

Spread sauce down the center of the dough only. Cover the sauce with 2–3 cups of the cheese and the pizza toppings, then cover with the rest of the cheese. Use a pizza cutter to cut strips along each side of the dough (even numbers on each side). Starting at the bottom, take each piece and cross, twist, and press the piece to the other side of the filling. Continue crisscrossing until your pizza is braided. Carefully place on a greased cookie sheet. If freezing, see directions below. Otherwise, bake at 400° for 18–20 minutes or until golden brown. After it is removed from the oven, brush the top with melted butter and sprinkle with garlic salt and parmesan cheese. Cut into pieces.

Freezing directions: Wrap in plastic wrap and then aluminum foil. Best results if this one is thawed completely before baking. Include butter, garlic salt, and parmesan cheese with this meal.

Pizza Roll-Ups

A fun way to serve pizza—kids love anything that can be dipped.

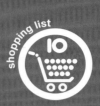

shopping list

- 20 loaves frozen bread dough
- 5 lbs. shredded mozzarella cheese
- 20 (15 oz.) cans tomato sauce
- Abt. ¼ cup Italian herb seasoning
- Abt. ⅔ cup fresh parsley
- assorted pizza toppings

2 loaves frozen bread dough
2 cups mozzarella cheese
1 cup pizza sauce (to go on pizza)
3 cups pizza sauce (for dipping)
toppings (pepperoni, sausage, ham, pineapple, black olives, etc.)

Pizza Sauce:
2 (15 oz.) cans tomato sauce
1 tsp. Italian herb seasoning
1 Tbsp. fresh parsley

Thaw dough. Using both loaves together, roll into a 14×24-inch rectangle (¼-inch thick). Spread 1 cup pizza sauce mixture on dough. Sprinkle cheese evenly on top of sauce. Top with your choice of toppings.

Roll up lengthwise like a jelly roll and cut into twenty-four 1-inch slices.

If freezing, see directions below. Otherwise, spray cookie sheet with non-stick spray and place rolls about 1 inch apart. Bake at 400° for 8–12 minutes. Heat sauce in a saucepan, and serve as a dipping sauce.

Freezing directions: Place roll-ups on a cookie sheet sprayed with non-stick cooking spray, and flash freeze. When frozen, place 12 roll-ups in a freezer bag. Freeze the dipping sauce in a separate freezer bag.

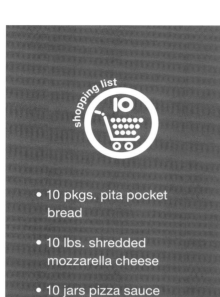

- 10 pkgs. pita pocket bread

- 10 lbs. shredded mozzarella cheese

- 10 jars pizza sauce

- desired pizza toppings

Pocket Pizza

These make great lunches as well as quick dinners!

1 pkg. pita pocket bread
1 lb. mozzarella cheese
1 jar pizza sauce
desired pizza toppings such as pepperoni, Canadian bacon, pineapple
    tidbits, or whatever your family likes.

Cut pita bread in half and open up to make a pocket. Fill with 3–4 tablespoons pizza sauce, ⅓ cup shredded mozzarella cheese, and desired toppings. If freezing, see directions below. Otherwise, microwave for 1 minute.

Freezing directions: Wrap in a paper towel or commercial deli paper. Place 6 wrapped pizzas in a gallon freezer bag. Include 12 pocket pizzas per meal. Microwave 1½ minutes from frozen.

Ravioli Casserole

Lasagna flavor, without the work!

1 jar spaghetti sauce
1 pkg. (25 oz.) frozen cheese ravioli, cooked and drained
2 cups small curd cottage cheese
4 cups shredded mozzarella cheese
¼ cup shredded parmesan cheese

Spread ½ cup of spaghetti sauce in 9×13 pan. Layer with half of the ravioli, 1¼ cups of sauce, 1 cup of cottage cheese, and 2 cups of mozzarella cheese. Repeat layers. Sprinkle with the parmesan cheese. If freezing, see directions below. Otherwise, bake uncovered at 350° for 30 to 40 minutes or until bubbly. Let stand 5 minutes before serving.

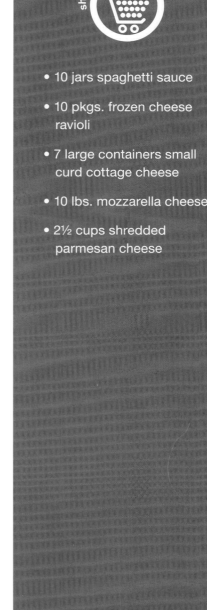

shopping list 10

- 10 jars spaghetti sauce
- 10 pkgs. frozen cheese ravioli
- 7 large containers small curd cottage cheese
- 10 lbs. mozzarella cheese
- 2½ cups shredded parmesan cheese

Freezing directions: Place in a disposable aluminum pan. Cover with foil and freeze.

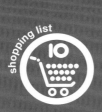
- 20 cups prepared spaghetti noodles

- 10 cups shredded parmesan cheese

- 30 eggs

- 3¾ cup butter

- Abt. 1 cup parsley flakes

- Abt. ¼ cup salt

- 20 cups ricotta cheese

- 5 tsp. Italian seasoning

- Abt. 2 tsp. pepper

- 10 lbs ground beef

- 20 cups spaghetti sauce

- 10 cups mozzarella cheese, shredded

Spaghetti Pie

Better than plain old spaghetti—your kids will ask for this one!

Crust:
2 cups prepared spaghetti noodles
½ cup shredded parmesan cheese
3 beaten eggs
3 Tbsp. melted butter
1½ Tbsp. parsley flakes
½ tsp. salt

Filling:
2 cups ricotta cheese
½ cup shredded parmesan cheese
½ tsp. salt
½ tsp. Italian seasoning
dash of black pepper

Top Layer:
1 lb. ground beef, browned
2 cups spaghetti sauce
1 cup mozzarella cheese, shredded

Combine all ingredients for crust. Spread mixture around sides and bottom of a 9×13 pan to form a crust. For filling, mix all ingredients together and spread over noodles. Mix beef and spaghetti sauce and pour over the filling. If freezing, see directions below. Otherwise, bake at 375° for 40 minutes. Top with mozzarella cheese and put back in the oven until melted. Let sit for 5 minutes before cutting.

Freezing directions: Slightly undercook spaghetti noodles. Place in a disposable aluminum pan and cover tightly with plastic wrap and then with foil. Include a bag of the mozzarella cheese to top with during the last 10 minutes of baking. When making this in bulk, do it assembly line style. Prepare the crust, place in all the pans, then the filling, etc. If you bake this from frozen, keep covered for the first half of baking.

Stromboli

Great Friday night finger food!

1 loaf bread dough
8 slices deli ham, thinly sliced
20 slices pepperoni
8 slices provolone cheese
2 Tbsp. shredded parmesan cheese
1 cup mozzarella cheese
1 tsp. garlic powder
1 tsp. dried oregano
¼ tsp. dried parsley flakes
¼ tsp. pepper
1 egg yolk, beaten

Let dough rise until doubled. Roll loaf into a 15×12-inch rectangle. Arrange meats and cheeses down the middle of rectangle dough. Sprinkle each layer with spices. Fold dough around meat and seal pressing dough together on seams and ends. If freezing, see directions below. Otherwise, place seam-side down on greased baking sheet. Brush with beaten egg yolk. Bake at 375° for 25 to 30 minutes. Let stand 5 minutes before slicing. Slice loaves on a diagonal.

Freezing directions: Wrap loaf with plastic wrap and then foil. Make a note on preparation instructions to beat an egg and brush it on the loaf before baking.

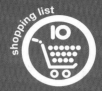

shopping list

- 10 loaves bread dough

- Abt. 3 lbs. thinly sliced deli ham

- Abt. 4 lbs. pepperoni

- 4 lbs. sliced provolone cheese

- 1¼ cups parmesan cheese

- Abt. 3 lbs. shredded mozzarella cheese

- 2½ Tbsp. garlic powder

- 2½ Tbsp. oregano

- 2½ tsp. dried parsley flakes

- 2½ tsp. pepper

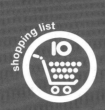

Yummy Spaghetti Casserole

Don't let the name fool you—this casserole has no tomato flavor.
Even our pickiest eaters loved this one!

1 can cream of mushroom soup
¾ cup milk
½ tsp. pepper
seasoned salt to taste
½ tsp. sugar
1 (12 oz.) pkg. angel hair pasta
2 cups sour cream
garlic salt to taste
½ cup parmesan cheese
1½ lbs. cheddar cheese
1 onion, minced
1½ cups bread crumbs
1 cup Ritz crackers, crumbled
½ cube butter

Blend together soup, milk, pepper, seasoned salt, and sugar. Set aside. Bring 4 quarts water to a boil. Add the pasta; remove from heat and let stand until pasta becomes pliable (about 10 minutes). Drain. Mix pasta with sour cream. Put in a greased 9×13 pan. Sprinkle with garlic salt and parmesan cheese. Top with cheese, then onions, and then bread crumbs. Pour soup mixture over all. Sauté cracker crumbs in butter until golden. Sprinkle over casserole. If freezing, see directions below. Otherwise, bake at 325° for 1 hour or until casserole is bubbly.

Freezing directions: Slightly undercook noodles. Place in a disposable aluminum pan and cover tightly with foil. If cooking this from frozen, keep covered the first half of baking.

Index

About the Author

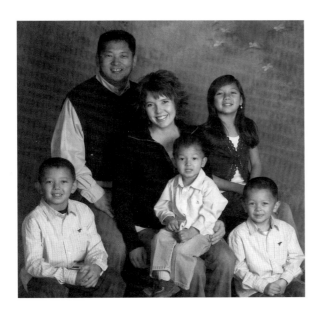

Suzie Roberts is one of those busy mothers who knows how challenging (not to mention boring!) putting dinner on the table night after night can be. She started her own Make-Ahead Meal Group in 2004 and became such a believer in this method of cooking that she decided to share her success with others. She continues to come up with creative and fun ways to give her more time to spend with family and friends. Suzie lives in Perry, Utah, with her husband, David, and their four children, Kyra, Kuen, Tatem, and Bryson.

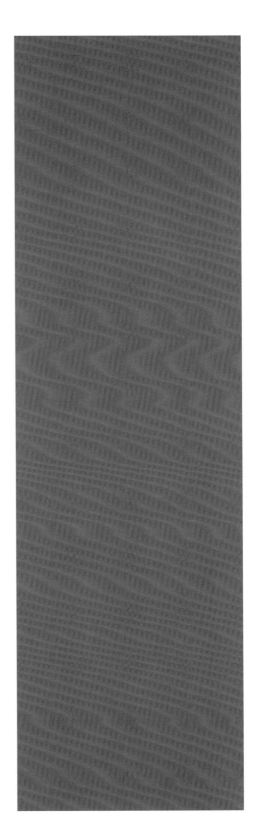